Smile de Look

georgen

on you

Dr. Paul

Praise for *Age with Style*

The mouth is beginning of the digestive tract. It tells you so much about how the digestive and immune system are working, from if you are adequately producing sufficient amount of digestive enzymes to properly digest food, to having a healthy microbiome and being well-hydrated. When a dentist looks at the oral cavity in a holistic, functional way, he/she can learn so much about what is going on inside one's body and begin to understand the root cause of disease. They have an opportunity to educate their patients on their overall health. Dr. Nammy Patel has developed an amazing program on how to take care of the whole person and make a huge impact both on patients' health and the environment. She cares deeply about her patients. Do read this book, for it is the future of health and the practice of dentistry. It really is an extraordinary guidebook whose time has come.

—Payal Bhandari, MD
Integrative Holistic Physician and Medical Director
www.sfadvancedhealth.com

Most people go to the dentist because they "have to." They go for a cleaning and check-up, and hope that nothing is wrong. But a biological/functional, holistic dentist has so much more to offer than just cleanings, fillings, and a nice smile.

Many years ago, dentistry was removed as a specialty in medicine and given its own class of doctors. However, the oral cavity is not separate from the rest of the body.

In this book, Dr. Patel has done a wonderful job telling you why she has so much more to offer every person than just the routine you may have come to expect during your dental visits. She has laid out why dentistry is an essential part of everyone's health journey and has made it easy and straight forward to find the answers to the questions you probably never knew how to ask.

Before your next visit to your dentist, this book is a must read. It will allow you to ask your dentist about some of the specific issues she raises.

You will be happy and satisfied.

—Dick Thom, DDS, ND
American Center for Biological Medicine, Scottsdale, AZ

Dr. Patel offers us a concise, easy to read and inclusive guide to holistic dentistry, and she's done it exceptionally well. It covers the tools you need to navigate your own health while creating a deeper understanding of biological human needs and how they can be met with the right dentist.

This is not a coincidence. Dr. Patel's cultural roots in traditional India combined with her scientific mind and commitment to detail are a powerful formula. This is also not a coincidence. She wants us to benefit from the latest scientific data, but she also wants us to not lose sight of the biggest picture of ourselves. Her patients are surrounded by the most biologically friendly environment possible and receive inspired dental techniques. But they also get warm neck pillows and conversation about the totality of their life and dreams.

If you want to know how your dental health is impacting your overall health, read this book. If you want to know and benefit from the latest best practices for holistic dentistry, read this book. If you just want to spend some time with a healthcare professional who has dedicated her life to the art and science of healthy living, read this book. Know that you are in the hands of someone who will guide you through the things you need to know to better understand your body, your health and how holistic dentistry can get you where you need to go.

—Tiffany Hunter, PhD
Healing for People, Co-founder and Clinic Director

AGE WITH STYLE

Namrata Patel, DDS

Age
—*with*—
Style

YOUR GUIDE TO
A YOUTHFUL SMILE &
HEALTHY LIVING

ForbesBooks

Published by ForbesBooks, Charleston, South Carolina.
Member of Advantage Media Group.

ForbesBooks is a registered trademark, and the ForbesBooks colophon is a trademark of Forbes Media, LLC.

Printed in the United States of America.

10 9 8 7 6 5 4 3 2 1

ISBN: 978-1-946633-59-0
LCCN: 2018958898

Book design by Megan Elger.

This publication is designed to provide accurate and authoritative information in regard to the subject matter covered. It is sold with the understanding that the publisher is not engaged in rendering legal, accounting, or other professional services. If legal advice or other expert assistance is required, the services of a competent professional person should be sought.

Advantage Media Group is proud to be a part of the Tree Neutral® program. Tree Neutral offsets the number of trees consumed in the production and printing of this book by taking proactive steps such as planting trees in direct proportion to the number of trees used to print books. To learn more about Tree Neutral, please visit **www.treeneutral.com**.

Since 1917, the Forbes mission has remained constant. Global Champions of Entrepreneurial Capitalism. ForbesBooks exists to further that aim by bringing the Stories, Passion, and Knowledge of top thought leaders to the forefront. ForbesBooks brings you The Best in Business. To be considered for publication, please visit **www.forbesbooks.com**.

To God, Source, Universe,
who made all this possible.

TABLE OF CONTENTS

FOREWORD

Do you want to age with style? Is your smile and how you look and feel as you age important to you? Look no further—this is the book for you.

As a naturopathic doctor practicing functional endocrinology in San Francisco, I am an expert in natural medicine, anti-aging and hormone balancing. I focus on treating the whole person by looking for the underlying imbalance—the root cause of disease. The majority of my patients are women going through menopause or are postmenopausal. As we age and our hormones decline, it can affect our bone health and gums which can affect our teeth and ultimately our digestive systems and overall health.

I often utilize bioidentical hormone replacement therapy (BHRT) as a primary treatment of anti-aging medicine. BHRT focuses on the slowing down of the human aging process as well as optimizing biological performance through identifying and treating hormonal biochemical imbalances and deficiencies. With the use of BHRT, we can replace deficient hormones with natural hormones that are identical in chemical and molecular structure to those produced by the human body. Preventing bone loss is one of the major uses for BHRT in my practice. I believe that diet and nutrition are the cornerstones of your health, digestion starts in your mouth and having healthy teeth and gums are the first part of a healthy system.

I first met Dr. Nammy Patel in 2008 when we collaborated on an open house to educate our mutual patients on health and wellness. After working together, I came to realize that she was much more than just a green dentist—she was a true advocate for natural medicine. I have been enthusiastically referring my patients to Dr. Patel ever since then. I have a long personal history of dental issues myself and have worked with Dr. Patel on removing my amalgam fillings and correcting bruxism—grinding of the teeth that can cause damage to teeth and gums. She is by far the most compassionate and holistic dentist I have worked with.

As a patient of Dr. Patel's, I know firsthand that her approach to your dental health comes from a deep understanding of the body's functions and knowledge of natural medicine. Dr. Patel has taught me how important gum and bone health are in the aging process and how they go beyond a pretty smile.

One other thing—Dr. Patel is a leader in her industry, and a pioneer in the field of functional, holistic dentistry. Like me, she realizes that true health and wellness requires a balanced approach to medicine. She treats the whole person and understands the importance of prevention. She looks at the underlying causes of gum disease and bone loss by asking the question: *Is it your diet, digestion or hormonal imbalance?* She is dedicated to helping her patients optimize their health from the inside out.

Dr. Patel wants your teeth to last for a lifetime, she wants you to be comfortable and have a healthy and pretty smile. To do this, she works closely with her patients and encourages them to investigate further into their health. It is from this functional, holistic dentistry philosophy that she approaches every patient. She understands that your health is reflected not only in your smile but in every aspect of your system. Dr. Patel is the perfect person to write a book about holistic dentistry and its connection to overall health.

I highly recommend this book to all my patients, friends and family who want to look and feel their best for years to come. Dr. Patel gives a well-written and easy to follow guide on how to age with style.

Dr. Erika Horowitz, ND
founder of Dr. Erika Horowitz Life. In Balance.
San Francisco, California

ACKNOWLEDGMENTS

This book is for my father, who gave up school at the age of nine to provide for his brothers and sisters. My mother, who gave me a life worth living. My brother Ashish (his name means "blessings"), who passed away and has given me the vision of a legacy for the Ashishkshama non-profit center in India. My sisters Tejal and Kalpana who have supported me unconditionally.

INTRODUCTION

I was born in the living room of my home in Dharotha, India. We lived in a village of eight houses and my mom milked the buffaloes for fresh raw milk daily. We farmed our own organic vegetables in our back yard. As a child, I remember being given turmeric for a cough, and eating ginger and garlic to boost my immunity. My parents immigrated to the United States when I was five years old, bringing their ancient culture, with its strictures and proscriptions, with them.

I loved the benefits of ayurveda—traditional medicine—and the family values that came with East Indian culture, but it was a traditional culture, one in which women simply didn't have career aspirations or go to college, much less to medical school. My parents' plan for me was the same as their parents' plan for them had been: I would have an arranged marriage and get busy having babies! If I worked, it would be in a limited role in the family business. My primary job was to run my household and care for my husband and children.

But that wasn't my plan. An inner feeling haunted me—I guess you would call a gut feeling or my internal compass—telling me I was on this planet for a bigger purpose.

I have always been "different" in our family. As a child, my sisters would play with barbie and cabbage patch dolls. I chose GI Joe and Transformers action figures because they were leaders fighting for a greater cause. They were interested in bettering society. While many girls were fantasizing about their wedding, I would take electronics apart and rebuild them.

Initially, I studied premed and planned to become a neurologist. I was fascinated by the miraculous way the brain works. A lot of my friends were studying to be dentists, but dentistry was not interesting to me. Working in the mouth? Yuck! No thank you! I knew too that people viewed dentists as "merely" dentists, not as real doctors. But one summer afternoon, I had an experience that completely changed the direction of my life. I was in an organic chemistry class and one of my friends in the predental program asked if I'd like to join her as a volunteer at a dental clinic—St. Mary's Dental Clinic in Stockton, California.

The clinic served the underserved, most of them poor farmworkers with no access to medical or dental care. And it was just as gross as I'd expected it to be. But somehow, as I assisted the doctors, I got past the challenges of blood and spit buckets to a point where I was really present. I was holding people's hands as they got their shots, and comforting them, and they were so grateful. They were afraid, and they didn't know what to expect. But they could see that I was there to help them—to just be present with them, and that was profound for them—and for me. I felt a powerful heart connection. Most of all, I felt needed; I was serving, I was useful. I felt like I mattered. In a small way, I had a positive impact on their lives.

As time went on, I got to know the patients. They began asking for me and bringing me little gifts—candy bars or some fruit they'd picked—to thank me for being there for them. I felt I'd found my calling; I wanted to help people, and this was the way to do it. That was a turning point for me. I left neurology and went into dentistry. In the years since that realization, my ideas about what good medicine is have solidified, largely through my own experiences—and led me to embrace functional, medicine-based holistic dentistry.

What Is Functional Medicine-Based Holistic Dentistry?

According to The Institute for Functional Medicine, "Functional Medicine is a systems biology-based approach that focuses on identifying and addressing the root cause of disease. Each symptom or differential diagnosis may be one of many contributing to an individual's illness…For example depression can be caused by many different factors, including inflammation. Likewise, a cause such as inflammation may lead to a number of different diagnoses, including depression. The precise manifestation of each cause depends on the individual's genes, environment, and lifestyle, and only treatments that address the right cause will have lasting benefit beyond symptom suppression."[1]

What specifically is functional, holistic biologic dentistry? It's the opposite of common dental culture, which is simply "drill and fill." Functional holistic dentistry is looking at and addressing the *underlying cause* of problems. When I explain it to a new patient, I share my own experience as an illustration:

---

1   "The Functional Medicine Approach," What is Functional Medicine? The Institute for Functional Medicine, https://www.ifm.org/functional-medicine/what-is-functional-medicine.

When I was in dental school, I'd study until midnight, and then be up at five o'clock in the morning to get to my class at six. In retrospect, it's to be expected that this stressful lifestyle took its toll. I was perpetually exhausted. I wondered if I had low thyroid levels, but every time I was tested my physician said, "It's on the low end, but it's no big deal. You're fine. It doesn't mean anything." So I let it go and just kept moving forward. After all, the doctor knows best, right?

I finished school and started my practice. My stress increased as I worked long hours, wearing many hats. My exhaustion got worse. Finally, my body said, "Enough!" and I had a breakdown. I hit the bottom. I could not get out of bed in the mornings because I was just too tired. I now know it was adrenal fatigue. But at the time, my doctor couldn't or wouldn't diagnose me. I was hooked on caffeine and sugar, stuck in a cycle of ebb and flood: high energy, low energy, high energy, and low energy. It started to feel normal to me, but of course, it wasn't. At one point, I even thought I was depressed. *Why didn't I want to go out with my friends?* I felt like the life had been sucked out of me.

I finally roused myself to take action, because clearly I could not continue in this way. My stress was still there, and my regular medical doctors still wouldn't treat me for the adrenal problems I knew I had. Instead, they offered me anti-anxiety drugs! Really? All I wanted was for them to focus on finding the real cause. When I showed them that my fingernails were dry, brittle and cracked frequently, which is symptomatic of both thyroid issues and low iron, they suggested I drink more milk.

With my health in the balance, I had to take measures in my own hands. I found practitioners who would treat the underlying causes of my ongoing problems. I started seeing an Ayurvedic practitioner and worked with a nutritionist. I adopted a vegan nutrition program, eating raw foods, and being more mindful about how much water I drank. After being on my raw vegan diet for four months, I started to regain my energy. I felt like I had gotten my life back. I was able to practice with joy again.

The Functional Dentistry Difference—Going Deeper

In functional, holistic dentistry, we look at four different things:

1. How do we make your teeth functional so you can chew properly?

2. How do we make sure you're comfortable?

3. How do we make sure your teeth last a lifetime?

4. And how do we make sure your teeth look good?

We're discovering ways to contribute to your overall body health focusing on prevention. We're committed to using the most natural available materials in your treatment. We look at the underlying causes for gum disease and cavities: is it your diet, hormonal changes, or acid reflux?

Much of what I've learned wasn't taught in dental school. I've had to seek it out myself. Fortunately, the dental school I attended had a problem-based learning program that encouraged independent thinking and not rote memorization. I was trained to be a critical thinker. Problems were posed to us, and we were expected to go and dig up the evidence for the solution we proposed.

An example: Mrs. Richardson comes in and reports she has trouble swallowing. What could the cause be? As a student, I had to come up with a list of potential causes. Then a few days later, I would be given more information about the patient's symptoms that helped me narrow down the actual cause. It was a great educational system. It gave me the intellectual tools I'd need to work with real patients whose underlying medical issues might not always be easily identifiable. I learned how to efficiently do differential diagnoses on patients with conditions that were commonly overlooked. I looked for solutions that a pill was not going to fix.

When I graduated from dental school, I began the process of interviewing and working at dental offices. Honestly, what I saw made me sad. Services were too often dictated by what insurance companies would or would not pay. Issues that could and should have been treated early on were left unaddressed or undertreated. The only rationale seemed to be that they could bill more if the problem got worse. Most of these practices weren't even owned by dentists; corporations owned them. In order to maximize profits, the directive was to see as many patients as possible in the shortest possible time. None of this aligned with my values. There was also tremendous waste generated, which challenged me. I am devoted to the Jain faith and it's engrained in me to conserve all resources. I literally cannot waste anything—it's just not in my DNA.

Those interactions confirmed what I knew: I had to make a change. I wanted to practice dentistry that was good for people and ecologically responsible. I looked at the whole individual. I wanted to give them tools that would prevent further health deterioration. And I wanted to do it in an eco-friendly way, not just recycling, but also in terms of the materials we use.

This is a key distinguishing factor in my practice. Some dentists will say, "We're green because we recycle." That is only one layer: It's also making sure you have BPA-free night guards, or that you have ionic air filtration in the office. It's using only composites that will not cause an increase in estrogen. If you're using vitamin E, is it gluten-free vitamin E? Those details matter to me, because they matter to my patients.

And my practice is mission-driven. I'm a deeply spiritual person. I believe that I'm here in this life for a purpose. I am here to help people live longer, healthier, more joyful lives. When I started Green Dentistry fourteen years ago, I was a trailblazer. But now I'm seeing that progress is needed in the medical and dental fields. We need to focus on treatments that provide long-term solutions. The band-aid approach to treatment is no longer acceptable, and we must look for the root cause of problems. Whew—this is a change that's long overdue!

> I am here to help people live longer, healthier, more joyful lives.

This book is meant to change the way you *think*—not just about the importance of going to the dentist. But beyond that, this book is about how living a healthy lifestyle plays in your ability to live your best life. I get it—going to the dentist probably isn't the highpoint of your day. Even thinking about it makes some people uncomfortable, with needles, drills, and often a big bill at the end of it. It's worse when you have to contend with dentists who don't seem to hear you, or who are not as tuned into what you're feeling as they should be.

But that's not me, and not my practice. We are wholly patient-centered. Our goal goes beyond helping our patients keep their teeth; we want to make sure they're not only looking good but feeling good too. We do everything we can to make the experience pleasant, welcoming, and comforting; we treat you as an individual, not an appointment. We share what we've learned with you, so that you're empowered to make the best possible choices for your health.

That begins with learning—and I hope that what you read here informs, enlightens and inspires you to make the changes in your lifestyle that will help you on your journey to healthy living and a beautiful smile.

Take a moment to reflect…

Where are you in terms of your dental health? The condition of your mouth is a bellwether of your overall physical health, so pay attention to what it and the rest of your body is trying to tell you.

- How do you feel in general? Do you wake up tired?
- When you brush or floss, do your gums bleed? Do your gums look red and puffy?
- When you eat ice cream or have a cold drink, do you feel pain in your teeth?
- Do you sleep comfortably through the night, or do you frequently awaken?
- Have you been told that you snore?
- Do you suffer from migraines?
- Do you notice that your gums are receding?
- Does your jaw joint "pop" when you open your mouth? Do you experience jaw discomfort when you take a big bite of something?
- Are you able to chew comfortably, or do you have sore spots you habitually avoid?
- Are there white spots on your fingernails?
- Do you regularly experience mood swings?

- Are there dark circles under your eyes?

- Are you pregnant, or aware of having any hormonal imbalance?

- Is your mouth often dry?

- Are you taking any medications?

- What medical conditions exist in your family history?

- What dental problem did your parents and grandparents have?

- Does going to the dentist make you anxious? Do you avoid seeing a dentist because of your fears?

- Are you happy with your current dental practice?

- Would you like to slow down the aging process?

If you're curious, keep reading.
If you have any questions,
give us a call at 415-433-0119.

CHAPTER 1

Healthy Mouth, Healthy Body: Symptoms and What They Mean

For many years, even in the dental profession, it was assumed that your oral health had only a tangential effect on your overall health. We now know better: poor oral health, along with the resulting gum disease, *releases bacteria into our systems that create many life-threatening and potentially life-ending diseases and disorders.* Among these are:

- Heart disease

- Stroke

- High blood pressure

- Diabetes

- Obesity

- Emphysema

- Hepatitis C

- Alzheimer's Disease

- Arthritis

- Vitamin deficiencies

- Shortened lifespan

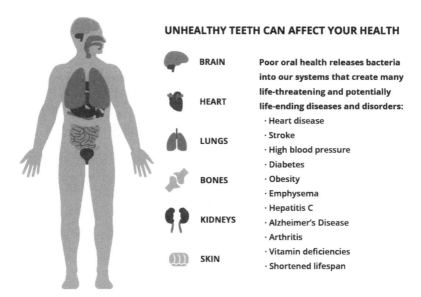

UNHEALTHY TEETH CAN AFFECT YOUR HEALTH

BRAIN

HEART

LUNGS

BONES

KIDNEYS

SKIN

Poor oral health releases bacteria into our systems that create many life-threatening and potentially life-ending diseases and disorders:

· Heart disease
· Stroke
· High blood pressure
· Diabetes
· Obesity
· Emphysema
· Hepatitis C
· Alzheimer's Disease
· Arthritis
· Vitamin deficiencies
· Shortened lifespan

The microbiome of our mouths includes over two hundred species of bacteria, some of which are helpful and some of which are harmful. Those good bacteria support health, just as those living in our gut do. Bad bacteria cause problems that go far beyond the mouth. When those bad bacteria are allowed to flourish in your mouth—when you're not flossing and brushing or having regular cleanings, as you should—your body is forced to expend a lot of energy and resources in fighting them. The result is an overwhelmed immune system. The same thing happens with your gut. An overgrowth of bad bacteria there leads to problems related to the gut that include decreased immune response.

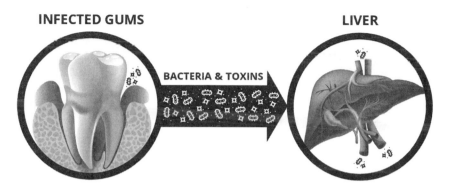

INFECTED GUMS   **LIVER**

BACTERIA & TOXINS

Bacteria and other poisonous toxins enter your general circulation through diseased gum tissue and infect the rest of your body!

Periodontitis (Gum Disease) is now linked to a variety of other health concerns including: Heart & Lung Disease, Alzheimer's Disease, Stroke, Diabetes, Colon Cancer, Obesity, and Premature Births

The reality of the human body is that it's not built to last forever; it's designed to disintegrate. Yes, we are designed to die. We are machines that are designed to fail over time, and the only way to slow down that inevitable degeneration is by preventative methods. For your teeth, this means flossing, brushing, and seeing your dentist at least twice a year. It also requires a healthy diet, sleep, exercise, meditation, and controlling your stress levels. Equally essential is making sure your hormones and your sugar levels are regulated. The mouth isn't separate from the rest of your body. It's part of the larger system, so whatever is happening in your body will be reflected in your oral health, and vice versa. When we're out of balance, bad bacteria can get a foothold and spread through the body in the blood stream, creating and spreading inflammation.

The story I always like to share is about my good friend Jack. I have known Jack for ten years now. Jack was a high-profile CEO, and very outgoing, always entertaining, traveling, and making deals happen. He was a busy guy, so it was hard for him to get to the dentist. I had warned Jack about the connection between gum disease and heart disease, but he shrugged it off. After all, he was only forty-five. He'd say, "Doc, you're a dentist, right? I see a cardiologist and everything is fine."

One day, I got a call at the office. It was Jack, who told my assistant his call was important.

"Hey, Jack! It's been a few years, how are you?" I asked.

He replied, "I could be better."

I said, "What's going on?"

"You wouldn't believe it. I had a heart attack!"

I like to use the kitchen analogy: if you don't sweep your kitchen floor every day, crumbs and dirt will build up, and it's going to attract bugs and vermin. Pretty soon your kitchen's overrun with them. Similarly, when poor hygiene allows bad bacteria to get a foothold in your mouth, they multiply—and every time you swallow them, they're moving down into all your body systems. Ick! A minimal amount isn't a problem, but when they get out of control, they overwhelm your body. When they get into your gut, your body uses energy to fight them off. It can't do its regular job of breaking down the food you eat that is supposed to give you energy. Bad bacteria in the body over a long period of time also cause hormonal problems (more about this in a later chapter).

The inflammation that began in your gums as gingivitis (or in its later stages, periodontitis) starts to move through your bloodstream and gets to the valves of your heart. This inflammation then leads to hardening of the arteries, and now, it is harder for the blood to circulate to the heart.

How Gum Disease Gets Started

The process works like this: Plaque, a sticky film made up of soft bacteria, attaches itself to your teeth and starts hardening. Hardened plaque becomes tartar. As they reproduce, the bacteria release acid and the acid attacks the gums and teeth. This process takes about six months to build up, which is why you must have your teeth cleaned twice a year. However, if you have a health-compromising condition—for example, you get lots of infections, have an autoimmune disorder, a hormonal disorder, dry mouth, active gum disease, or you take antidepressants, are pregnant, have diabetes, or are predisposed to cavities, you should have your teeth cleaned *every three months.*

Why are people so flakey about taking care of themselves and their oral hygiene? Even my own patients will dutifully follow the prescribed schedule of visits, exams, and cleanings for a while and then slack off because they're (a) so busy and/or (b) aren't in any actual pain, so it's easy to just put it off. The saying "Out of sight, out of mind" is relevant here.

But here's the thing: we are always going to have saliva, so we are always going to have bacteria. Even if you feel great and look great, those bacteria are multiplying in your mouth and damage is being done. Yes, you had a thorough cleaning. Yes, you're good about your oral hygiene, but not staying focused on the care of your mouth will cost you more in both time and money, later. *The need for care doesn't change, so your lifestyle has to change to accommodate the care you need.*

How do you know if you've got potentially dangerous bacterial levels in your teeth and gums? One sign is waking up with bad breath, or with a bitter taste in your mouth. If you have either of these symptoms on a regular basis, it's time to get your checkup! Probably, you're not flossing at night, and you should be. Bacteria love a dry breeding ground, and your mouth is a dry breeding ground when you're sleeping. Bacteria take that opportunity to multiply. Whether you're using dental floss or a WaterPik, *make sure you use it before you go to bed.*

Other symptoms of bacterial buildup include discolored teeth, swollen gums, or blood in your spit when you brush. A sharp pain in your teeth when you drink something hot or cold is a sign of trouble you shouldn't ignore. Waking up with general pain in your teeth and/or gums is a loud message that it's time to take better care of your mouth.

If you fail to nip this in the bud, it will lead to a whole cascade of negative consequences for your health. For one thing, if your teeth are giving you pain, you're going to avoid eating foods that are hard to chew, or you will underchew the foods you do consume. Leafy greens are the classic example. They're a critical part of a healthy diet. If you can't properly chew and digest them, you're starving your body of those essential nutrients, and if your gut is too busy fighting off bad bacteria to properly process what you do eat, you're going to miss out on many of those nutrients as the food passes through. You will be eating but not get the essential nutrients out of what you eat.

The Hormonal Connection

A hormonal imbalance—too much estrogen, thyroid or progesterone in the body—can be a cause of gum disease and dental caries (cavities). Estrogen levels are generally higher than they should be in both men and women, especially due to genetically modified soy and corn, and stress. Increased amounts of estrogen mean increased amounts of bacteria. As bacteria grow, they release acid that lowers the pH of the mouth, which softens and dissolves the enamel outer layer of the teeth and speeds the growth of bacteria. Even though you may be brushing, flossing, and going to the dentist, these bacteria are growing faster than they're supposed to. You can stop this by addressing the underlying condition through supportive therapies, and by cleaning the gums in a specific way.

Okay, time to tell the truth: What's standing between you and good dental care? What is causing you to let your oral health slide?

In my practice, *fear* is the number-one reason people don't get the care they should.

Nancy is a good example of that: sixty-five years old and recently retired, she had a bad experience with a dentist as a child, and even all these years later, the dental phobia that experience had created was powerful enough to keep her from getting the care she needed. She had not been to the dentist in over forty-five years. When a painful emergency finally brought her into my office, she had a great deal of bone loss. I think the only thing that kept her teeth in place was the tartar! I was able to help her, but treatment was much more extensive (and expensive) than it would have been if she'd been taking care of herself. I will talk more about the genesis of dental fear in a later chapter, and how a caring practitioner can help you to deal with it. It definitely stops many people from getting the care they need.

The other big concern I hear is about the cost of dentistry—and yes, dentistry is an investment. Science has proven that keeping your teeth adds an extra ten years to your life. Isn't that a great investment and one worth the effort of maintaining healthy teeth? Some say it's expensive. However, it's not nearly as expensive as it becomes when you avoid the simple maintenance that could prevent expensive fixes down the line. Do you neglect to change your car oil and do scheduled maintenance on your car? You probably do not, because your car represents a significant investment of your resources. You know that letting needed upkeep slide will wind up costing you far more in repairs. Your teeth are even more valuable than your car in terms of your health and happiness. If you doubt that, imagine doing without them. If you fail to take care of them, that's exactly what you will be doing!

Youth Is No Protection against Gum Disease

I believe that the most unaware patients are those in their twenties. Many just don't take care of their oral health with the same discipline they bring to getting to the gym every other day, or making time for morning yoga class. After all, nothing hurts and they look good. Even if their dentist warns them that something's dangerously wrong with their bite, or that there's a crack forming in a tooth, they're likely to shrug it off and use that as a reason to avoid going back to the dentist.

STAGES OF GUM DISEASE AND POCKET DEPTH

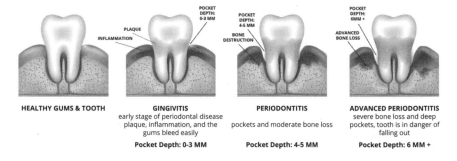

HEALTHY GUMS & TOOTH	GINGIVITIS	PERIODONTITIS	ADVANCED PERIODONTITIS
	early stage of periodontal disease plaque, inflammation, and the gums bleed easily	pockets and moderate bone loss	severe bone loss and deep pockets, tooth is in danger of falling out
	Pocket Depth: 0-3 MM	Pocket Depth: 4-5 MM	Pocket Depth: 6 MM +

Unfortunately, when that compromised tooth gives way, or their gums start bleeding, they finally come to the dentist, and what could have been fixed easily now requires much more extensive repair or replacement. It doesn't take long for damage to be done. In as little as a year and a half to two years, neglect can create an avalanche of issues. Some of the issues will be difficult if not impossible to fix. Often, I look at the damaged and sometimes unsalvageable teeth of patients in their fifties and wish I could have helped them thirty years earlier. Sadly, the damage has been done. Basically, if you don't see your dentist for two years, you're already compromising your health. If you skip visits for five years, you're going to see some bone loss. Ten years without professional dental care and you're almost certain to have severe bone loss.

The problem with bone loss is that you can't feel it happening. As you get older, your bones become less dense and more fragile. That is what osteoporosis is, why we tend to get shorter as we age, and why older people are more likely to break bones when they fall. Unfortunately, unhealthy bacteria in the mouth hasten the process of disintegration in the bone supporting your teeth, and then your teeth get loose and fall out. There's not much that can be done to stimulate bone growth once that happens. I'll talk more about the relationship between aging and tooth loss later on, but the short version is that you can hold on to those teeth much, much longer if you prevent bone loss with good habits that diminish bacterial growth.

Bottom line: Our bodies are designed to age and, ultimately, to die. Mortality is a given, but you can diminish and significantly slow down the effects of aging if you pay attention to your oral health. Let it slide, and everything else will surely slide with it.

FAQs on Oral Hygiene

Q. Should I invest in a Waterpik, or is flossing enough?

A. If you're willing to take the time to do a thorough job, flossing is fine. If you're not going to do it right, get a Waterpik. I'm all about gadgets when they work. Just make it simple. Make sure you've got the pressure turned up high enough to really get in there, and that you're following the directions for use. You can even add a spoonful of hydrogen peroxide to the water in the well to help in the bacteria-banishing efforts. And floss *before* you brush, not after.

Q. Electric or old-fashioned hand-powered toothbrush?

A. Electric toothbrushes work the best because they hit your teeth with fifty-thousand pulsations per minute and that's faster than Superman could brush! People with a receding gum line need to be careful and use their weaker hand to brush and go easy, because they tend to brush too hard. One gram of pressure is all you need to apply in brushing your teeth. One gram of pressure is a soft touch. The pressure has zero impact on the effectiveness of the cleaning; it's the length and thoroughness of the mechanical action that removes bacteria. You need to brush twice a day, regardless of the tool you use.

Q. Besides keeping my teeth clean, is there anything else I can do to stop the growth of harmful bacteria?

A. *Oil pulling* is a useful antibacterial therapy you can do at home. Using coconut oil, swish it around in your mouth for about ten to twenty minutes (longer is better). The bacteria that cause problems such as gingivitis, bad breath, and plaque will naturally adhere to the oil. When you're done, spit it into the trash (not the sink because coconut oil can harden and form clogs). Please note that while oil pulling can be useful as part of a regimen of good care, it does *not* take the place of regular professional cleanings. *Oil pulling does nothing to reverse the damage* *bacteria may already have done.* Once established on your teeth in the form of plaque, bacteria have to be scraped off, and no amount of oil will budge them.

Q. What about oral piercings?

A. Get them out of your mouth! Piercings will break your teeth because the metal constantly hits the enamel and the enamel is a brittle structure like crystal. A tongue piercing will chip your teeth, and a lip piercing will cause gum recession because the metal constantly abrades the gum tissue.

Q. Is vaping a problem?

A. The more we know about vaping, the less harmless it looks. As far as your teeth are concerned, vaping causes dry mouth and can encourage the buildup of bacteria and gum disease. Smoking does the same thing. Both of them will also discolor your teeth. Why do it?

Your Turn

What's Your Oral Care Quotient (OCQ)?

I brush my teeth ...

1. When I think of it—usually in the morning .
2. Twice a day, morning and night.
3. Two to three times a day—morning, after lunch, and before bed.

I floss...

1. Honestly? Never.

2. When I think of it—a couple of times a week.

3. Flossing is part of my daily routine.

I go to the dentist a for professional cleaning ...

1. When I can make time for it: every couple of years.

2. Once a year.

3. Twice a year or more.

My gums bleed ...

1. When I brush.

2. Only when I floss.

3. My gums don't bleed.

My attitude to going to the dentist is ...

1. I prefer to wait until I have to go. I'm busy, and who likes going to the dentist, anyway?

2. I go once a year, or I try to. Care is expensive!

3. I make time and set aside the money to go to the dentist, just as I make time for physicals. It's essential to my health.

Score

(Add up the numbers of the answers you chose.)

5–8: a dangerously low OCQ. Your habits are threatening your health. Change them, and become a better steward to your body. You only get one!

9–12: not terrible. You have plenty of room for improvement. Reread this chapter and look for ways to change your habits for the better.

13–15: You're way ahead of the curve! Good for you, and keep it up.

If you're curious, keep reading.
If you have some questions,
give us a call at 415-433-0119.

CHAPTER TWO

The Inflammatory Response

In the previous chapter, I talked about the damage that bacteria in the mouth cause throughout your body via inflammation. Let's dig a little deeper into what the inflammatory response is and what it does.

Inflammation is your body's response to injury, a way in which it tries to protect itself. This is a naturally occurring phenomenon, designed to work for you, but it does damage when it becomes a chronic condition. When you get a cut or a bruise, you've probably noticed that the area around that injury becomes reddened and warm. That's because your immune system has sent out mediators (cytokines) to protect the area from infection. A very similar thing happens when you have an internal infection, such as pneumonia. When you're injured or ill, this inflammatory response works to fight infection and to keep it from overwhelming your system, but when it goes into overdrive, it causes more problems than it solves. The example I like to use is when you're in a traffic jam, even though you're not getting anywhere, your car's engine is still running, so the gas is being used up, and you might even run out of fuel before you get where you need to go. The same happens with inflammation: when the body is under attack and focused on fighting off the infection, its resources are used up and little energy is left for healing and proper function.

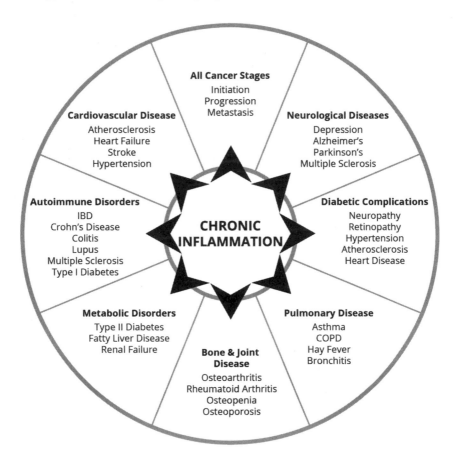

There are five signs of inflammation. The first is *rubor* (redness): as soon as bacteria hit your body, your blood vessels dilate so the white blood cells can travel more swiftly to the injury site. The second sign is *tumor* (swelling): that increase in vascularity (dilation of the blood vessels, associated with rubor) causes an increase of fluids rushing into the injury site, which in turn causes swelling around the injury. The third sign is *calor* (heat): increased blood flow to the wound site causes heat. The fourth sign is *dolor* (pain): the swelling and stretched pain receptors cause pain. The fifth sign is *functio laesa* (loss of function): injury impairs cell function. Inflammation itself falls into two types: *acute* and *chronic*. Acute inflammation happens in response to an injury or illness. Body tissue quickly resolves the condition when it becomes functional again. In other words, the body heals. But *chronic inflammation* means your body is suffering from a long-term infection or damage. It's constantly tasked with fighting off that infection. Examples are toxins from cigarette smoke, or the buildup of fatty plaque inside your arteries that causes atherosclerosis. Chronic inflammation could be described as acute inflammation on overdrive. It's a continuous response to infection that ultimately exhausts the body's resources. It arises when acute inflammation goes unresolved and tissue function is not restored. This results in functional loss and the death of cells.[2]

Chronic Infection in the Mouth

As I discussed in the previous chapter, your mouth hosts a whole naturally existing population of bacteria, both useful and harmful. When the body suffers a trauma of some kind, or a long-term illness, or if you suffer from autoimmune disorder, these bacteria will overgrow. The body will send its foot soldiers—the cytokines I mentioned earlier—and proteins to fight off this infestation. At that point, you see the initial signs of inflammation, rubor (redness) expressed in bleeding gums and gingivitis. If you're on a six-month cleaning schedule with your dentist, that next cleaning may not come

---

2   Ravinder Nagpal, Yuichiro Yamashiro, and Yuichi Izumi, "The Two-Way Association of Periodontal Infection with Systemic Disorders: An Overview," *Mediators of Inflammation*, December 2, 2015, http://dx.doi.org/10.1155/2015/793898.

quickly enough to prevent the onset of periodontitis and the loss of bone that entails.

Because this is chronic inflammation, it's defined by types of defense mechanisms that are different from those of acute inflammation. In the same way that crimes are addressed by jurisdictionally different law enforcement agencies from local police to the FBI, depending on the severity of the crime, when inflammation becomes chronic, our bodies deal with it through different "jurisdictions." *Tumor necrosis factor* (TNF) is one of our "first responders," produced during the acute phase reaction by activated macrophages. *Interleukins, prostaglandins,* and *proteinases* work together to kill off the bad bacteria. *Monocytes,* produced in the bone marrow, are the precursors to *macrophages,* which surround apoptotic cells and pathogens and produce immune effector molecules. In healing wounds, circulating *monocytes* also enter the tissue, becoming fibroblast-like cells called *fibrocytes.* All of these enter the fray, fighting those bacterial "criminals."

When you get a cleaning every six months, your dentist gets rid of the bacteria causing this response. When you miss a few visits, you will need a deep cleaning to address the chronic inflammation that's produced by those inflammatory mediators in your gum tissue. Meanwhile, however, macrophages and fibroblasts are damaging the tissue, breaking away the underlying bone structure that holds your teeth in place.

The damage doesn't stop there. When you swallow, you're putting those bacteria into play in your bloodstream, where they can attach themselves to your arteries. This causes atherosclerosis, or thickening and hardening of the arteries, because bacterial plaque is building up inside them, and as it's building up, your body's trying to fight it off. Over time, this plaque narrows the arteries. Eventually, an area of plaque can rupture; blood cell fragments (platelets) will stick there, forming blood clots that can break free and lodge in your heart, stopping the blood flow and causing a heart attack. The various bacteria linked to gum disease, among them, *P. gingivalis*, *tannerella*, *forsythells*, and *Prevotella intermedia*, are found in about 40 to 50 percent of the carotid arteries of people living in the United States.[3]

When my patient Derek came into the office seven years ago, he explained that he'd been under a lot of stress, going through a divorce and dealing with custody issues. He was forty-two years old, and it had been two years since his previous dental visit.

During my exam, I found he had bleeding gums, with a distinct keto odor. That set off alarm bells. I told him I was concerned that because of this stress, his age, and that telltale keto odor, he probably had periodontitis associated with diabetes. I asked him if he had had any lab work done recently, and when he admitted he hadn't, I urged him to see his doctor.

Three weeks later, he came back to the office and told me he'd been diagnosed with type 2 diabetes. I sent him to a nutritionist, and after meeting with her, he decided to go raw and vegan. Now, seven years later, he's doing much better—and he's much more diligent about getting to the dentist!

Diabetes and Inflammation

It's long been known that diabetics have an increased risk of gum disease. That makes sense because when you're diabetic, your body is already on overdrive, which puts you at heightened risk for infection. *But it's also true that people who have gum disease are more likely to become diabetic!* Tumor necrosis factor (TNF), which, you'll recall,

---

3 American Society for Microbiology, "Gum disease bacteria may cause heart disease," ScienceDaily, May 18, 2014, https://www.sciencedaily.com/releases/2014/05/140518164339.htm.

is produced during the acute phase of an inflammatory reaction by activated macrophages, also creates insulin resistance, the cause of type 2 diabetes.[4]

Respiratory Disease

It's not surprising that the bacteria growing in your mouth get into your ears, nose, throat, and lungs. Just as those bacteria can get into the arteries and cause problems, the same bacteria can create inflammation when they get into your lungs. When they're inhaled, your body's emergency response system goes into self-protection mode, which causes tissue damage. The bacteria most closely linked to respiratory issues are *Psuedomans abroginosa* and *Staphylococcus aureus*, and the tissue damage they do over the long term is linked to chronic obstructive pulmonary disease (COPD), which is a lung disease characterized by the chronic obstruction of lung airflow that interferes with normal breathing. COPD *is not fully reversible.*

Inflammation and Pregnancy

How is gum disease related to pregnancy? First, pregnant women are at greater risk for gum disease because of hormonal changes and increased blood flow. This can lead to what's called pregnancy gingivitis: swollen, red, and tender gums that bleed easily when brushed or flossed. Untreated, this can lead to periodontitis or even loose teeth. This is probably the basis for the old saying, "A lost tooth for every child." Fortunately, good oral care can prevent that unhappy outcome. If you're pregnant or think you might be, tell your

---

4 J. Garcia-LemecA and Sandra P. Farsky, "Hormonal Control of Inflammatory Responses," *Mediators of Inflammation* 2, no. 3 (1993): 181–198, http://dx.doi.org/10.1155/S0962935193000250.

dentist. Get those regular cleanings without fail because untreated gum disease can also present multiple challenges to your developing baby's health. Also, take your multivitamins because the embryo's tooth buds start developing after twenty-eight days of gestation.

Advanced periodontitis and chronic inflammation have been definitively linked to premature birth and low birth weight in babies.[5] They've even been associated with preeclampsia.[6] When a woman's body is ready to give birth, it releases hormones that start the labor process. One of these hormones is oxytocin, produced by the hypothalamus plus the prostaglandins, which stimulate the uterus to contract. When a pregnant woman has gum disease, that inflammation triggers an increase in immune response, which, in turn, spurs the production of prostaglandins as well as TNF, and the cytokines interleukin 1 and 6. These can cause the uterine membrane to rupture, triggering early contractions and premature birth.

Diseases Linked to Inflammation

Inflammation's disruption of normal hormone production can create a whole range of health consequences, from mild to devastating. I'll talk more extensively about hormones and their impact on both oral and overall health in a subsequent chapter, but in the context of inflammation, it's important to note its impact on the hormones responsible for normal bodily function—in this instance, cortisol and estrogen. When your body is stressed, as it is by inflammation, it responds by producing too much cortisol, which leads to the

5   Rajiv Saini, Santosh Saini and Sugandha R. Saini, "Periodontitis: A risk for delivery of premature labor and low-birth-weight infants," *J Nat Sci Biol Med* 1, no. 1 (Jul–Dec 2010): 40–42, https://doi.org/10.4103/0976-9668.71672.
6   Ben-Juan Wei et al., "Periodontal Disease and Risk of Preeclampsia: A Meta-Analysis of Observational Studies," *PLoS One* 8, no. 8 (August 2013): https://doi.org/10.1371/journal.pone.0070901.

production of excess estrogen, kicking up the inflammatory response another notch. When your body is stressed, it's on hyperdrive, constantly firing signals, which can spur autoimmune disorders such as rheumatoid arthritis or lupus.

My friend Ana has her own business and is a busy mom. Her level of cortisol and estrogen increased, which caused her to have irregular periods and to develop fibroids. We first noticed her bleeding gums during a cleaning, which led us to learn that she suffered from estrogen dominance. As she continued to work with the naturopath, we also discovered she had celiac disease.

Interestingly, older cultures have long been aware of the health threat of inflammation and have found ways to treat it. While they didn't understand the science behind bacteria in the mouth, the effects of inflammation on the body were evident. In ancient India and the Middle East, for instance, they brushed their teeth with the bark of the meswak tree, whose natural antibacterial properties fought gum disease.[7]

How Do We Fight Inflammation in the Mouth?

It can't be said too many times: brush, floss, and get regular cleanings. I recommend oil pulling, described in the previous chapter, and also rubbing coconut or sesame oil into your gums.

I'll talk about dealing with the problems caused by stress a little further along, but it's important to note here that changing your lifestyle to minimize stress is not only going to decrease inflammation but will also lengthen your telomeres, the DNA component tied to longevity. Reducing stress is really mostly a matter of creating good

---

7   Hilal Ahmad and K. Rajagopal, "*Salvadora persica* L. (Meswak) in dental hygiene," *The Saudi Journal for Dental Research* 5, no. 2 (July 2014): 130–134, https://doi. org/10.1016/j.sjdr.2014.02.002.

life habits: Exercise half an hour or longer a day. Get enough sleep, a minimum of eight hours a night. Practice meditation and deep breathing. All of these practices help your body to de-stress and to repair itself. Keep hydrated. Most adults don't drink enough water. Eat properly, and get enough of the necessary vitamins and minerals to support your immune system to help you heal.

Excessive amounts of any hormone naturally produced by the body can also create imbalances that favor bacterial growth. The pituitary gland releases certain hormones. They go through the hypothalamus, which releases a certain number of hormones in response. Basically, these hormones tell your body what to do, regulating the menstrual cycle, going bald, and so on. Too much of any hormone—for example, estrogen—stimulates the growth and propagation of bacteria. Thyroid imbalances can cause the same problem. Monitoring your hormone levels is essential to good health and good oral health.

Another stimulus to bacterial growth is your diet. If you're eating too much sugar or too many carbohydrates or snacking too frequently, you're feeding the bacteria in your mouth. I've seen the idea of grazing throughout the day put forth as a healthy alternative to three square meals a day. I can tell you, from an oral health perspective, that it is a disaster because you're basically turning your mouth into a bacteria buffet line.

Dry mouth, a naturally occurring phenomenon when we get into our fifties and beyond, is another big contributor to bacterial overgrowth. Dry mouth is also a common side effect of antianxiety and antidepressant medications. *Saliva fights off bacterial growth,* thanks to the antibodies it contains. It helps keep the mouth in balance. In its absence, bacteria reproduce much more quickly and are also able to adhere to teeth more easily. Rough surfaces in the mouth are also a handy breeding ground for bacteria. Fillings that aren't polished off, for instance, offer a foothold for bacteria to stick. The presence of certain metals in the mouth, including those found in amalgam fillings, also spur bacterial growth.

You prevent inflammation in your mouth by consistently attending to your oral hygiene. There's no reason for you, as an otherwise healthy person, to suffer from gum disease! While other things going on in your body can change the balance to favor bacterial growth, so much can be accomplished—or prevented—just by regular brushing, flossing, and visits to the dentist.

FAQs on Inflammation

Q. I'm switching from an IUD to birth control pills. Is that going to screw up my hormonal balance and create inflammation?

A. Since the hormones in birth control pills effectively mimic the changes the body experiences in pregnancy, it's important to let your dentist know that you've started taking them. Again, it's a question of taking effective preventative measures via good first-line hygiene practices and professional care. There's no reason your teeth will suffer if you stay on top of those.

Q. What are good ways to deal with dry mouth?

A. First, cut back on, or eliminate, the things that can make it worse, such as caffeine and antihistamines. Stay away from mouthwashes that contain alcohol, which is also drying, and if you smoke or vape, stop doing so. Try products that mimic saliva, such as sprays or rinses containing xylitol, or chew xylitol gum to stimulate salivation, keep a water bottle close to you, and stay hydrated, taking sips throughout the day.

Q. What are the best oils to use for oil pulling or gum massage?

A. Unrefined, organic, cold-pressed oils are best. You can use coconut or sesame oils (my favorites) or sunflower or olive oil. People also use avocado, walnut, cardamom, and many other oils.

Your Turn

- Do you eat multiple times during the day? Are you eating sugary or starchy snacks?
- Are your teeth extra sensitive to cold or heat?
- Are your gums puffy and swollen, or red?
- Is brushing or flossing painful?
- Do you see your dentist every six months, or more often if recommended? (Note: averaging doesn't count! Consistency is what matters.)

For women:

- Is your period regular?
- Do you sleep soundly at night?
- How would you rate your daily stress level? How do you mitigate it?
- Have you experienced a weight gain?

For men:

- Are you experiencing hair loss?

If you're curious, keep reading.
If you have some questions,
give us a call at 415-433-0119.

CHAPTER THREE

The Truth about Amalgam Fillings

Chances are that if you're reading this book, you're at least tangentially aware of the storm of controversy in the holistic health-care world around the dangers of amalgam fillings. In this chapter, I'll talk about the issues with amalgam fillings, why it matters whether or not you've got them, and what you ought to do if you have them.

What Is Amalgam?

Dental amalgam is a mixture of metals. About half of its weight is made up of a powdered alloy of silver, tin, and copper, with the other 50 percent being elemental mercury. Sometimes minute amounts of zinc, palladium, or indium are included too. Mercury is used because it keeps the other ingredients pliable long enough to press the compound into a tooth. Once it hardens, it's strong enough to withstand the forces put on it in biting and chewing.

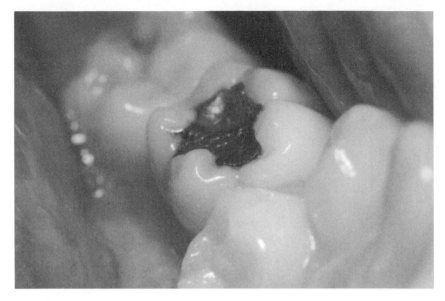

There's no problem with mercury when it's just sitting there as part of the amalgam. The problem arises when you chew, or brush your teeth. The abrasion creates heat and causes the mercury to off-gas. Chewing gum is especially bad for this. Even drinking a hot beverage releases mercury vapors in your mouth. Those vapors get swallowed and go into your body, where they're stored—and that creates significant health hazards, because we're talking about a known poison. This process is called *bioaccumulation*.

What Does Mercury Do?

Mercury kills white blood cells as well as T-cells, which we need to fight off infection and bacteria. So it lowers immunity. Once in the stomach, it deposits itself in the *mesenchyme*, the single-layer cell lining of body cavities. Bacteria exposed to mercury become resistant to antibiotics.

Common symptoms of mercury exposure range from fatigue, moodiness, and the inability to concentrate, to lack of confidence and depression. Some people will experience headaches; some will become arthritic, and others will develop more serious autoimmune disorders such as multiple sclerosis. There is no such thing as a "safe" level of exposure; mercury is a poison, even in minute doses.

The age at which any of these kinds of symptoms show up, and whether or not they do, depends on the individual, but youth isn't necessarily any protection. Ari is a young man of twenty-four who came to me with a mouthful of amalgam fillings he'd had since he was a child—and a litany of illnesses. His bones hurt, and he was getting arthritic. He suffered with chronic sinus infections and allergies. For someone his age, he was a mess, and I had to agree that at twenty-four, he shouldn't have been dealing with autoimmune diseases, poor health, and arthritis. He'd done some research on his own and suspected the problem might be mercury from his fillings, and he wanted them out. Could I do that?

I could and did. We removed all those amalgam fillings, and he began to see steady improvements. His arthritis is now cleared up, the allergy attacks have been reduced by about 80 percent, and he's getting back the kind of energy a guy his age should have.

Other health issues are related to mercury build-up too. Research has shown that rats exposed to mercury develop Alzheimer's-like symptoms,[8] and mercury also kills sperm. Mercury inhibits zinc and manganese absorption, which is needed for sperm to swim, and it also inhibits the production of DNA in sperm. In women, it binds to proteins and becomes organic mercury, which is even worse because it denatures proteins and makes the metabolism dysfunctional. At the tissue level, mercury builds up in the hypothalamus and the pituitary gland, which are critical to health because they release the

---

8   Joachim Mutter et al., "Does Inorganic Mercury Play a Role in Alzheimer's Disease? A Systematic Review and an Integrated Molecular Mechanism," *Journal of Alzheimer's Disease* 22, no. 2 (October 2010): 357–374, https://doi.org/10.3233/JAD-2010-100705.

hormones that regulate the entire body, from heart rate to ovaries to testosterone to blood pressure.

If you're a woman of child-bearing age, you should know that the mercury you inadvertently consume is also a significant hazard to your developing fetus since mercury can also pass through the placenta. It can also enter a mother's milk. Studies of the effects of heavy metals including mercury suggest that they can be a factor in spontaneous abortion.[9] Mercury interferes with enzyme cytochrome P450, a critical liver enzyme that makes hormones (among them progesterone) and breaks down many medications.

Many of my patients are women in their childbearing years who are trying to get pregnant. One of them, Susan, was a beautiful, healthy woman of thirty-three who had been trying for about five years. She'd had several miscarriages and been unable to carry a child to term. She came to me and we looked at her mercury levels. We decided it was time to get the mercury out of her mouth and out of her system. Once I removed the amalgam fillings, she went through a detox program. Shortly after that, she got pregnant, carried her baby to term, and gave birth to a healthy child, who's now six years old.

Mercury in the heart causes oxidative stress, which means increased inflammation. Mercury vapor goes into the heart and brain, as well as the pituitary, thyroid, and adrenal glands where it blocks acetylcholine, a neurotransmitter that passes signals to the organs and tissues. Acetylcholine is really important because it tells the neurotransmitters what to tell the nerve cells in the body. Acetylcholine stimulates your vagus nerve, which controls the fight-or-flight response. When acetylcholine is blocked, the vagus can't deliver the message to your body. It dictates the beat of your heart.

---

9   Cecilia Nwadiuto et al., "Heavy Metals in Miscarriages and Stillbirths in Developing Nations," *Middle East Fertility Society Journal* 22, no. 2 (June 2017): 91–100, https://www.sciencedirect.com/journal/middle-east-fertility-society-journal/vol/22/issue/2.

It dictates how effectively your digestive system works, since food is moved through your intestines by contractions called peristalsis. Without it, nothing works as it's supposed to.

Mercury and Alzheimer's Disease

Alzheimer's disease, a degenerative disease of the brain, is the most common form of dementia and currently the fifth most frequent cause of death in the United States. It's a major public health crisis, and, as our population ages, is expected to increase exponentially.

This incurable and invariably lethal disease presents in seven stages. In the first, no decline in cognition is evident. The second stage is mild forgetfulness; previously simple things, such as remembering appointments or where you left your keys become more difficult, and you're likely to ask the same question multiple times, or make the same remark without remembering you've done so. Still, the symptoms may not be all that evident to those around you or to your doctor.

Increasing confusion and forgetfulness begin in the third stage; the names of people or things escape you, you have trouble thinking of the right word to use, and planning and organizing become impossible. In the fourth stage, you begin to have trouble doing simple math problems, will likely be unable to handle your own finances, and may forget not only short-term things such as what you had for breakfast, but details about your life history.

Fifth-stage Alzheimer's is when things really begin to go south. You may not remember how to dress appropriately, or recall your own phone number or address. In the sixth stage, your personality changes: you become moody, angry, and paranoid, forgetting even familiar people. You may wander off, and you will lose control of your bowels and bladder and require watching and a lot of assistance with the everyday functions of life. In the seventh stage, you're nearing death and can no longer communicate or care for yourself.

How does mercury fit into this? Mercury binds to acetylcholine, which is a neurotransmitter. Nerves have a scaffolding-like tubular construction, made up of microtubules that, in turn, make up tubulins. Picture this "nerve skeleton" as being like a railroad or a highway that allows the nerves to communicate. Mercury disrupts this movement of signals, stopping the tubulin from working, which kills that skeletal support and disrupts transmission of information along that highway. Picture a bridge collapsing between the two points you're traveling between; without that bridge, you either can't go from point A to point B, or you need to find an alternative route. This is the same kind of cellular damage we see occurring in Alzheimer's.

Let's be clear here, though. Not everyone who's exposed to mercury will develop mercury poisoning, much less Alzheimer's disease. To some extent, the disease is contingent on genetics, and the degree of exposure you have. Let's say for instance that you have a genetic marker for Alzheimer's, you're from a culture that consumes a lot of fish, and you've got a mouthful of silver fillings. Chances are that you'd be more likely to experience these mercury toxicity issues than someone without silver fillings, who doesn't eat fish. If we both had the same number of fillings, but I had no genetic predisposition at all, it wouldn't matter as much. It is really the mercury vapor released over time and stored in the body that is the issue.

Having a particular form of a gene called ApoE heightens your risk of Alzheimer's. The ApoE gene provides instructions for making a protein called apolipoprotein E. This protein combines with fats (lipids) in the body to form molecules called lipoproteins.

Lipoproteins are responsible for packaging cholesterol and other fats and carrying them through the bloodstream. Maintaining normal levels of cholesterol is essential for the prevention of disorders that affect the heart and blood vessels (cardiovascular diseases), including heart attack and stroke.

There are three different versions of this gene; the third one, ApoE4, increases your risk for developing late-onset Alzheimer's and may also cause early-onset memory loss. ApoE4 is associated with the protein clumps (amyloid plaques) found in the brain tissues of people with the disease, and it's believed that a buildup of these clumps is at least partly responsible for the symptoms of the disorder. About one in seven people have this gene. The problem is that ApoE4 contains sulfur, and mercury loves sulfur, so it binds to the sulfur group in the gene, preventing the gene from doing its job of clearing out the plaque clumps in the brain, so they build up.

Do You Have Mercury Issues?

What are some of the most familiar "tells" of mercury poisoning? Thyroid problems are very common among people who have a toxic level of mercury in their systems. People with mercury issues often get candida, a fungal infection that shows that your body isn't fighting off invaders as it should be. The cells that make up the mesenchymal layer, that single-layer cell lining of body cavities, stop functioning as they should, and their vital job of exchanging nutrients and waste is slowed or blocked. A common example of that is someone who can't hold chiropractic adjustments for a long time.

How Is Mercury Removed?

Your body will excrete mercury to some extent through the bowel and through the skin, which you can help along with saunas or Epsom salt baths.

Treatment with a salt of a chemical called *ethylenediaminetetraacetic acid* (EDTA) is used in what's called *chelation therapy* to treat mercury and lead poisoning because it binds metal ions to remove them from the body. The supplement *chlorella* is a detoxifier that binds to heavy metals and gets them out of the body. And vitamins A, D, E, and K, all antioxidants, will also help to remove mercury. It also helps to use a sauna, or steam room, to excrete the metal out of your body. Activated charcoal binds to mercury and helps with elimination.

Your first step should be to have those amalgam fillings removed before they can do any more damage to your system, and it's important to work with a dentist who has the experience and the skills to do this properly to avoid any further exposure to mercury in the process of having the fillings removed.

In my practice, I use the least amount of epinephrine (anesthesia) possible while making sure my patients are comfortable, and I use the least toxic form of anesthesia, one which goes into and out of their system very quickly.

When we're working on a tooth with an amalgam filling, we use the SMART protocol. The first step is to isolate the tooth using a rubber dam so that mercury vapor isn't released. Using copious amounts of water and suction to pull the vapor and any fragments out of the mouth, I make incisions in the filling that allow me to pop it out.

Once the mercury is out of your mouth, you can use the supplements I mentioned above to help speed the residual mercury out of your system.

FAQs on Amalgam Fillings

Q. What kinds of alternatives are there to amalgam fillings?

A. We use metal-free, mercury-free composite fillings that look great, blend in with the patient's tooth color and will last for years.

Q. If I have mercury in my fillings, does that mean I'm going to get Alzheimer's?

A. No. What we know about the factors influencing Alzheimer's disease is that they include a strong genetic predisposition, your diet, your lifestyle, and what toxins are in your environment. But mercury can play a part in tipping the scales toward getting the disease, as it weakens your defenses against the disease and promotes the buildup of the plaque in the brain associated with Alzheimer's.

Q. Can any dentist remove my fillings?

A. Any dentist *can*, but to avoid additional and unnecessary further exposure to mercury, choose a dentist who is experienced in the SMART protocols of removing fillings while protecting you from the vapors generated by the removal process. Why make the problem worse in trying to solve it?

Your Turn

Am I at Risk for Mercury Poisoning?

- How often do you eat the following fish, known to be high in mercury?

- □ Shark
- □ Swordfish
- □ Grouper.
- □ Chilean sea bass.
- □ Bluefish.
- □ Halibut.
- □ Sablefish (black cod)
- □ Spanish mackerel (Gulf) and king mackerel
- □ Fresh tuna (except skipjack)

- How many amalgam fillings are in your mouth? How long have you had them? The more you have and the longer they've been in place, the greater your exposure is.

- Do you live near a coal-fired power plant? Significant amounts of mercury exist in the air pollution created by these plants.

- Have you used a skin-lightening product manufactured in a country other than the USA? Many of these contain mercury.

- Have you got any of the symptoms or disorders associated with high levels of mercury in the system? These can include
  - □ Irritability or nervousness
  - □ Depression
  - □ Numbness
  - □ Memory problems
  - □ Physical tremors

- Difficulty in conceiving (both men and women), or in carrying a pregnancy to term
- Autoimmune disorders
- Mood swings, irritability or other emotional changes
- Insomnia
- Frequent headaches
- Weakness and muscle atrophy
- Loss of cognitive function

As the levels of mercury in the body rise, more symptoms will appear.

If you're curious, keep reading.
If you have some questions,
give us a call at 415-433-0119.

CHAPTER FOUR

Hormones and Your Health

I've talked a little about hormones and their effect on your oral health in previous chapters, but you may still be operating under the assumption that if you're not experiencing some very specific, situational hormonal upheaval, such as pregnancy, you're off the hook as far as hormones are concerned and can safely skip this chapter. Wrong!

The experience of a patient of mine, Suzanna, is typical of the cascade of health issues a hormonal imbalance can create. In her mid-thirties, Suzanna is a powerhouse, type A go-getter who came to me with jaw pain, complaining about tightness in her jaw and overwhelming exhaustion. She explained how stressful her life was and had been for many years, all made worse by the death of her father: "I don't know what's wrong with me, but I just can't seem to get back on track." Examining her, it was clear to me that she was grinding her teeth like crazy, and her bleeding gums were a signal that something was out of whack. The grinding didn't surprise me. It's a classic symptom of stress overload, and her work and life were certainly stressful. What did surprise me was her exhaustion. This former dynamo had had trouble just getting out of bed in the morning.

When I talked to her about it, she revealed that her medical doctor had examined her and determined her problem was depression, exacerbated by her father's death, and he prescribed antidepressants. Fortunately, a visit to a naturopath uncovered the underlying issue: stress-related hormonal imbalance and high cortisol levels that mimicked depression in their physical effects. Her body was breaking down because of the stress, and she'd hit the wall thanks to adrenal fatigue.

We took care of her, got her gums cleaned up, and fixed her bite. I recently saw her for her post-op exam. She's feeling amazing now because I gave her some jaw exercises she could use to help alleviate the muscle tension that she has. As a woman in a service-oriented profession where I give to everyone all day long, I understand how easy it is to get caught up in the habit of putting out more energy than you have on a daily basis, and I shared some of my own de-stressing practices with her.

It's easy to blame her medical doctor for misdiagnosing her, but it really comes down to the difference between that school of thought and holistic medicine. Holistic practitioners dig for the root causes rather than treating the symptoms. Frankly, because of the way health care is today, doctors just don't have the time to ask the questions that need to be answered, because so little time can be spent with a patient. However, her doctor should have looked deeper, in this case, because antidepressants wouldn't have done a thing to fix her adrenal stress and the subsequent hormonal imbalance. In fact, the antidepressants would have caused dry mouth and increased gum disease and cavities.

How Hormones Work

Reader, be advised that this section may get a little dense at times, but hang in there! Knowledge is power, and understanding how your body chemistry works is essential to making smarter choices that support healthy living.

To understand the importance of hormones in the regulation of your bodily systems, you need to know how they work. Hormones and their receptors are like a lock and a key. The hormone receptor is the lock, and enzymes or chemical messengers are the key. A hormone attaches to a hormone receptor and makes something happen. On a cellular level, the hormone effectively goes to the cell, tells the DNA to make messenger RNA (mRNA), which processes the formation of protein. The protein is the building block, the product that tells your skin tissue to repair itself, for instance, or your body to have a period.

For example, the antidiuretic hormones are ADH and aldosterone, which regulate the water in the body. Let's say there aren't enough electrolytes in your body. The hypothalamus is signaled and puts the ADH hormone into the body, which signals the kidneys to retain water. Aldosterone, the main mineralocorticoid hormone, is a steroid hormone produced by the adrenal cortex in the adrenal gland. It tells the body to retain water by increasing sodium and potassium in the blood. Aldosterone responds to a decrease in blood pressure, versus angiotensin, which responds to an increase in blood pressure. If there's an increase in blood pressure, you have an increase in angiotensin, which tells the adrenal cortex to make more aldosterone. If you don't get enough hormones such as ADH, you'll drink a lot of water, but the kidneys won't be able to absorb it, so you'll suffer from dehydration, potentially even death.

Reproductive hormones in men and women give their bodies their baby-making marching orders. In the hypothalamus, FSH is the follicle-stimulating hormone and luteinizing hormone, both of which go to the testes or ovaries, respectively, functioning differently in each gender. In a man's testes, it gives the order to make testosterone. In a woman's ovaries, it gives the order to make progesterone and estradiol.

Glucose is regulated by *glucagon* in thyroid hormones *T3* and *T4*. When your sugar intake is increased, your level of insulin will increase because the purpose of insulin is to distribute the sugar. *Glycogen* is, basically, the stored form of sugar. Diabetes occurs when there's too much sugar in the blood, usually because your body's insulin isn't working properly. When there's a decrease in sugar, the glucagon tells the T3 and T4 hormones to come into play, and they take the glucose and make energy. When sugar is broken down in the body, it's used for energy. The T3 thyroid hormone (triiodothyronine) is the most active thyroid hormone. If you're hypothyroidic, you're not able to break down sugar efficiently, which is why people with that condition tend to be lethargic.

Calcium released from bone is regulated by the *parathyroid hormone*. Vitamin D is converted to *calcidiol* in the liver and then converted to *calcitriol* (the biologically active form of the vitamin) in the kidneys. Calcitrol is critical to bone health and oral health, since it regulates the blood levels of of calcium and phosphorus, which build bones and teeth. When the parathyroid hormone level increases, it starts leaching calcium and breaking down teeth, putting calcium in the blood. Vitamin D deficiencies will cause cavities.

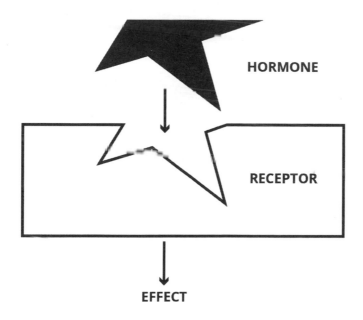

HORMONE

RECEPTOR

EFFECT

So Why Do You Need to Know This?

If you're like most of us in this pressure-cooker world, you're under an unrelenting physical assault of stress, both long-term and short-term stress, which plays havoc with your hormone balances.

Short-term stress causes that familiar "fight-or-flight" response, kicking up your blood sugar, increasing the flow of oxygen to your organs, and speeding up your heart rate. Obviously, this kind of reaction eats up a lot of your energy reserves. When you suffer from long-term, chronic stress, those resources and reserves are tapped to exhaustion, upsetting the body's hormonal balances. Chronic stress causes a big increase in cortisol and aldosterone, so you start experiencing a lot of energy breakdowns. Chronic stress prevents your metabolism from functioning properly, because your body is putting any energy it might have into converting glycogen into glucagon. It's the hormonal equivalent of having an unbalanced checkbook, or withdrawing funds from a retirement account ahead of schedule—not a good idea. Long-term stress creates inflammation and devastates the immune system. In terms of dental health, this can cause gingivitis, gum disease, and cavities.

Stress raises cortisol to levels that can decrease *osteocalcin* in bone, which, in turn, leads to the loss of calcium. Stress also causes an increase in blood pressure and disrupts the sex cycle by decreasing the level of *gonadotropin*, a hormone that is secreted by the pituitary gland and stimulates gonad activity. Stress decreases available growth hormones, and insulin, causing increased sugar in the body. It also causes hypothyroidism, which can cause, among other things, the TSH receptors to become defective. This impairs the production of T-cells, thereby damaging the immune system.

Remember my analogy of hormones and hormone receptors working together like a key and a lock? In this scenario, the lock becomes defective. Your body starts storing fat because of excess levels of cortisol and the carb- and fat-craving hormone leptin (leptin tells you you're hungry). Cortisol stops the breakdown of fat and increases *glycogenolysis*, the synthesis of new sugar. Excess cortisol also impairs the function of osteoblasts by decreasing *osteocalcin*, which is regulated by vitamin D. This can lead to bad bone health and weakened teeth.

Estrogen Dominance and Women

Estrogen dominance is defined as an excess of estrogen relative to the amount of progesterone in the body. This isn't just a woman's issue, by the way. Estrogen dominance occurs both in men and women and there are many things that can bring it on, as you will see below.

As we age, our bodies are supposed to manufacture less estrogen and less progesterone. Estrogen dominance happens when the drop in progesterone is greater than the drop in estrogen. That ratio is really critical because when there's too much estrogen, it causes a lot of issues, including bleeding gums and the breakdown of bone support. A decrease in progesterone, or a surge in estrogen, can cause this. It can cause other problems too. Estrogen builds the uterine lining and controls body fat, but it may also have a negative effect on thyroid hormones. Excess estrogen decreases your sex drive, causes blood clotting, and increases the incidence of endometrial cancer and breast cancer. *Progesterone* maintains the uterine lining. It uses fat for energy, is an antidepressant, helps thyroid function, normalizes blood clotting, protects the body from cancer tumors, and regulates blood sugar. These two hormones need to be in balance. In women, estrogen's primary role is to tell the uterus and the sexual organs to prepare the uterine lining for an egg. In both men and women, it affects skeletal growth through fat, protein definition, and electrolyte balance. Progesterone is a building block for *corticosteroids*, which we need to balance electrolytes, to regulate blood pressure, and to counter stress.

Women usually begin experiencing mild estrogen dominance symptoms in their mid- to late-thirties, with symptoms worsening over time as the gap between estrogen and progesterone widens. The ratio of progesterone to estrogen naturally shifts in women who are between thirty-five and fifty years of age: we see a 35 percent decrease in estrogen and a 75 percent decrease in progesterone.[10] This coincides with premenopause, perimenopause, and the onset of menopause and is part of normal aging.

---

10   Sara Gottfried, *Younger: A Breakthrough Program to Reset Your Genes, Reverse Aging, and Turn Back the Clock 10 Years* (San Francisco: HarperOne, 2017).

As noted above, men go through estrogen dominance as well. Estrogen in men plays an important role in the regulation of testosterone, several brain functions, bone health, skin health, libido, the cardiovascular function, and cholesterol. Typical estrogen dominance signs for men include

- Sexual dysfunction (low libido, decreased morning erections, decreased erectile function)

- Enlarged breasts

- Lower urinary tract symptoms associated with benign prostatic hyperplasia (BPH),

- Increased abdominal fat (can also be a symptom of low estrogen)

- Feeling tired

- Loss of muscle mass

- Emotional disturbances, especially depression

- Type 2 diabetes

Birth-control pills also create estrogen dominance: fooling your body into thinking you're pregnant so as to prevent conception causes the increase of estrogen.

Environmental estrogen such as that found in canned goods, commercially raised red meat plastics, soy beans, deodorant, and artificial sweeteners also increase your estrogen levels. Moreover, stress, as we've seen, causes adrenal fatigue, which increases estrogen. Chances are that if you're under a lot of stress, you're also not sleeping all that well, which taxes your adrenal gland too. Again, this isn't just a problem experienced by women; men suffer from it too.

Our Goal Is to Treat the Cause, Not the Symptoms

In my practice, I often see patients with symptoms that include bleeding gums and loss of bone. Sometimes I'll see an uptick in the formation of cavities because the body and the mouth have become more acidic. Gum disease is often an indication of estrogen dominance. Low progesterone is what eats away at the bone structure and decreases immunity, causing your gums to bleed.

The best way forward is to treat these issues with a deep laser cleaning, which has long-lasting effects in killing off those marauding bacteria. The cleaning is followed up with a maintenance program using a customized solution to prevent further bacterial buildup.

The body is a complex matrix of interconnected systems, each of which has an impact on the health of the whole organism. The key in diagnosing and treating hormonal imbalances is to look beyond the obvious (the symptoms) to the root cause, a process that's too often bypassed in traditional (allopathic) dentistry and general medicine.

If you suspect that stress is damaging your health, you're probably right.

FAQs on Hormones

Q. I'm expecting a baby. Should I skip dentist visits until she's born? I don't want to take any risks.

A. Absolutely not—and the reason is hormones. The hormonal changes your body undergoes during pregnancy actually make you more vulnerable to gum disease and tooth decay. This high hormone level causes more blood flow to the gums, which can make them swell, bleed more easily, and become inflamed. Regular and frequent cleanings become even more important now because your health affects your baby's health. Do tell your dentist that you're pregnant, and don't skip those visits. Make sure you're being extra vigilant with your oral hygiene at home too.

Q. As an older man, I'm feeling the effects of decreased testosterone on my libido and energy levels. How does this affect my oral health?

A. We're seeing research suggesting that low testosterone impedes the body's ability to build or maintain bones and teeth. A study done on castrated macaques showed that both the jawbones and teeth of the monkeys were less robust and strong than those of other males.[11] They also showed signs of much more severe periodontitis than other males.

Your Turn

- Have you noticed changes in how you're feeling, physically and emotionally?
- Do any of the following apply to you?
  - I just don't have the energy I used to have.
  - I think I'm depressed; I never feel like seeing my friends after work, because I just want to sleep.
  - I've gained ten pounds in the last year, but my eating habits haven't changed.

---

11   Qian Wang et al., "The Mandibles of Castrated Male Rhesus Macaques (*Macaca mulatta*): The Effects of Orchidectomy on Bone and Teeth," *American Journal of Physical Anthropology* 159, no. 1 (August 21, 2015): 31–51, https://doi.org/10.1002/ajpa.22833.

- I'm so much moodier than I used to be.
- I'm working out as much as I ever did, but I'm not getting the results I used to get.
- I used to really enjoy sex with my partner, but these days I'm just not interested.
- I'm always hungry.
- I never had insomnia before, but now I toss and turn all night.
- My gums are so sore and tender.
- Stress is wearing me down.

If any of these sound familiar to you, your hormones may be out of whack. Talk to your doctor or health practitioner about your symptoms and ask if testing can be done to uncover the cause. Don't take no for an answer. Ultimately, your health is in your hands, and you must be your own advocate.

If you're curious, keep reading.
If you have some questions,
give us a call at 415-433-0119.

CHAPTER FIVE

The Power of a Smile

What does a great smile say about you? Much more than you might think, and it has a surprising impact on how you're seen by others.

There are so many interlinked components to a smile and how we respond to it. First, it reflects our health. Are our teeth straight and white, or stained and crooked? Is our breath fresh or stale? When we smile, the condition of our mouth says a lot about our overall well-being because our body detoxes through our mouth.

There's also an emotional component to our smile because we so often show affection with our mouth—we kiss, we whisper, we nuzzle—and a beautiful smile is an invitation to get closer. A not-so-great smile, or one we hide, is off-putting—and makes us look less than trustworthy, which is definitely *not* sexy. Smiling is one of the love languages. Think of great family dinners where everyone at the table is laughing and smiling as food and stories are shared. A great smile says so much without speaking a word: "Come sit by me," or

"I'd like to know you better." A smile is an affirmation; it lets others know we are amiably disposed to them. A smile is a gift, something given freely, an act of generosity that warms the hearts of both the giver and the receiver. A smile is an act of service, something we do consciously to put others at ease. Smiling creates a sense of comfort and safety and takes away others' primordial fear of the unknown.

Our smile has a powerful impact on our self-esteem. Growing up being ashamed of our smile has an impact on how we interact with others. People who are uncomfortable with smiling will cover their mouth with their hand, clamp their lips together, or look down so that others don't see their teeth. In school, the boy whose teeth are crooked is less likely to raise his hand, speak up in class, or do well in class presentations. Teachers may mistake this reticence for ignorance or disinterest and give the child low grades because of it. When adults are ashamed of their teeth, they avoid interacting face-to-face with others, speaking up in meetings, and taking opportunities to network, all of which can have a negative impact on a career.

There's also a spiritual component to our smile, which is damaged when something so central to who we are makes us feel "less than," or unlovable. When we're able to smile and we look good, we feel good. It adds to our self-esteem, allowing us to be more present, more confident, less defensive, and more open.

Apart from how our smile makes us feel about ourselves, there's something else to consider; how do others see us? That matters because while we humans have always been appearance-conscious, in the last ten or fifteen years the bar has been set even higher. Remember when nobody had whitened teeth, other than newscasters and movie actors? Now most people do, to some degree, particularly in the upper echelons of the professional world. Have you noticed how rare it is to see ugly teeth in people at the top of their profession, or working in upper-level management, or in any position in which they deal directly with the public? That's not by accident. Research has shown that when you meet someone new, you gain your first impression of that person within a fraction of a second, and once made, that first impression is stubbornly resistant to change.[12] Since, not surprisingly, a smiling face registers as welcoming and honest, it shouldn't come as a shock that having good teeth makes a big difference in how that first impression stacks up.

My patient Liz, fifty years old, had worked at the same institution for five years but had never received a promotion. We gave her a full set of veneers, and three months later, she came back and told us that all her colleagues had said her energy had shifted: she was so much fun to be around and was always smiling—and she received a 15 percent raise!

In a 2001 study, researchers L. Harker and D. Keltner examined the relationship of positive emotional expression (smiles) in women's college pictures to personality, observer ratings, and life outcomes.[13] Women who smiled in their yearbook photos were more likely to rate themselves as competent, upbeat, and friendly. More to the point, those who looked at their photos rated the smiling women more favorably, and "expected interactions with them to be more rewarding; thus, demonstrating the beneficial social consequences of positive emotions." In other words, people looking at the women smiling in their photos liked them without ever having met them! Even more powerfully, when the researchers interviewed the smiling women

---

12 Society for Personality and Social Psychology, "Even fact will not change first impressions," ScienceDaily, August 5, 2018, https://www.sciencedaily.com/releases/2014/02/140214111207.htm.

13 L. Harker and D. Keltner, "Expressions of Positive Emotion in Women's College Yearbook Pictures and Their Relationship to Personality and Life Outcomes across Adulthood," *Journal of Personality and Social Psychology* 80, no. 1 (2001): 112–124, http://dx.doi.org/10.1037/0022-3514.80.1.112.

up to thirty years after those college photos had been taken, it was found that the smiling women had better life outcomes: higher levels of personal well-being and more successful marriages. Additionally, the researchers noted that "controlling for physical attractiveness and social desirability had little impact on these findings."

People make assumptions about your social class and income based solely on the appearance of your face, and the first thing they're most likely to notice about it is whether or not you're smiling, and how your teeth look, according to a study by R. Thora Bjorsdottir and Nicholas O. Rule at the University of Toronto.[14] In this study, undergraduates were asked to look at photos of peoples' faces (carefully stripped of other visible clues such as piercings and tattoos) and pick out those who were well-off from those who were not. Impressively they were right 68 percent of the time. The researchers found that the undergraduates based their assessment on people's mouths—specifically, smiling mouths. People who were smiling were generally seen as wealthier, and therefore more successful, than those who were not. Furthermore, the smilers were rated more likely to land a job than those whose faces were neutral.

Why do we respond to people in this way? I think it's because how we take care of ourselves signifies a lot about us, from income/class/status to a sense of responsibility. I know it sounds odd, but I'd never have a financial advisor whose teeth were all over the place. Why would I assume that financial advisors who don't take care of themselves would be on top of looking after my money? Maybe, they're broke and can't afford to fix their teeth, a bad sign for financial experts, or maybe those teeth are symptomatic of drug abuse. Yikes!

---

14   R. Thora Bjornsdottir and Nicholas O. Rule, "The Visibility of Social Class from Facial Cues," *Journal of Personality and Social Psychology* 113 (2017): 530–546, https://doi.org/10.1037/pspa0000091.

What happens when we don't smile? We're seen as less trustworthy, less attractive, and less warm. Do you remember that, for a while, all over the social media, there were photos of women who had what people called a "resting bitch face"? The fact is, we do look better when we smile, and we make those around us feel better too.

Now, we could make a good argument that snap judgments based solely on appearance are unfair and even unwise, but that's how our brains are hardwired to perceive others. Life is tough and it comes at us fast, but when someone smiles at us, it slows things down a bit; it gets us to take stock of the encounter; it brings us back to connecting and reciprocating with others, whether they are our child, husband, boss, or coworker. And did you know that the physical act of smiling itself is therapeutic for the smiler? The act of smiling activates the release of neuropeptides in the body that diminish stress. Neuropeptides allow communication among neurons related to the emotional state. The happiness-generating neurotransmitters—dopamine, endorphins, and serotonin—are all released by smiling, lifting mood, relieving stress, and even lowering the heart rate, while endorphins provide natural pain relief.[15] The kicker is, it doesn't matter whether your smile is from the heart or just an expression you've pasted on as a social gesture. Your body automatically reacts positively to the physical cue your smile sends your brain. Even if you don't feel like smiling, putting a smile on your face releases the chemicals that make you feel better.

On the other hand, if you're not smiling, you're shortchanging yourself on so many levels. For example, low self-esteem is powerfully bound to depression, and who needs that? We need to feel we belong.

15 Tara L. Kraft and Sarah D. Pressman, "Grin and Bear It: The Influence of Manipulated Facial Expression on the Stress Response," *Psychological Science* 23, no. 11 (2012): 1372–1378, https://www.ncbi.nlm.nih.gov/pubmed/23012270.

Feeling we're going to be rejected by our community because we don't look like them is damaging. I remember loving the character She-Ra when I was a little girl, but it was also tough for me to have her as a heroine, because she didn't look like me. I was a little brown-skinned girl with big teeth like Bugs Bunny's. How could I ever measure up to She-Ra? It was limiting. I know that as a child I felt shy about speaking. I felt ugly. I knew who I was, but I couldn't communicate that to the world, because I was too self-conscious, too much aware that I didn't look like others.

When people grow older and their teeth start to show their age, it can cause them to feel marginalized and to withdraw socially. They lose their smiles, or they can't eat properly, and so are likely to avoid social situations involving food. They're so focused on their embarrassment that it isolates them, even in a crowd.

Getting Your Smile Back Is Wonderful

One of the most satisfying things about my work is giving people beautiful smiles. Seeing those transformations—not just how the smile looks to others but also how the people with the beautiful smiles feel about themselves—is always special and unique.

One patient of mine is a chef, a dad of five, about forty years old, and a great guy. One day he told me, "I don't like my smile. I'm embarrassed about it." His teeth were yellow and chipped. They had white spots on them from having worn braces (and not taking good care of his hygiene when they were on). He described himself as feeling "dirty"—and he was tired of that feeling. We went for it: a full smile rejuvenation, with sixteen veneers. It was as if he'd dropped years off his looks, and his self-esteem soared as people reacted positively to his new appearance. That was ten years ago and his smile still looks great.

I'm very particular about the type of porcelain I use. Not every dentist is, but I know that high-quality materials are key to making those veneers last a long time. Sometimes, creating a beautiful smile requires more than one process or technology. I had a patient come to see me who very obviously had not been to a dentist in a long, long time. Bonnie's teeth were discolored and crooked. She explained that she came from a poor background and her parents didn't have the money to straighten her teeth. She'd been waiting for years to do something about it but was very shy and uncomfortable, embarrassed even to have them examined.

I put her into Invisalign aligners and the results were great. She was thrilled and told me she wanted to go with the full "Hollywood smile"—white and bright. I whitened her teeth with in-office whitening and then I reshaped some of the teeth with *enamelplasty*, a very easy and quick technique that lets me bring a slightly too-large tooth down a bit in size or shape to match the teeth around it. When the teeth aren't aligning properly, it's pretty common that one tooth will be shorter than the other or there'll be some jagged edges, and this lets us fix those little "mistakes." Once we evened them out, everything looked great.

Her transformation is something to see—not just her smile but her whole appearance, including the way she carries herself, and interacts with the world around her. She has a magnetic, life-loving personality that had been hidden behind her self-consciousness, and over the year and a half that we worked to bring her new smile into being, we saw that personality bloom. When she came to us, initially, she wasn't dating anyone and was clearly ill at ease with those around her. Within a few months, as the aligners did their work, she confided that she was "seeing someone" and was pretty happy about that. Her personal style, even her walk, proclaimed a new pride and sense of self: "I'm present. I'm happy. I'm comfortable with who I am." The biggest life journey is being comfortable with who we are.

Let's talk about some of the challenges your smile might be facing and the fixes we can do to make it better.

The "Gummy" Smile

Do your gums spoil your smile because they cover too much of your teeth? That used to require gum surgery with a scalpel, which is about as much fun as it sounds! But using a modern laser tool, we can move the gums up easily, a procedure that's nearly painless and can be done in half an hour.

Chipped, Jagged, or Uneven Teeth

Enamelplasty, as I mentioned, is a very quick and effective way to buff minor irregularities off your teeth: jagged edges, little chips, or even taking a little off a tooth that's slightly longer than the tooth next to it. It's a small adjustment but can make a surprising difference in your smile.

Bonding and Veneers

If you've a front tooth with a chip that's too large to buff out, we can repair it with bonding, using a tooth-colored composite, but if we need to make a more dramatic change to the size and shape of a tooth, we use veneers. These are thin shells of porcelain or composite resin that are customized to fit on top of your tooth, a little like a press-on nail. Good veneers have a tooth-like translucence that makes them look completely natural. Not-so-good veneers can look like a row of Chiclets. Veneers resist stains and can hide chips and stains.

Worn-down teeth or spaces between teeth that shouldn't be there can also be covered with veneers.

The process for making veneers requires taking a mold of your teeth, and sending it to a lab. We use that to make temporary veneers that look like the real thing so the patient can try them on and see how they look and feel. Adjustments can be made at that point so that the final product will be perfect. Good-quality veneers will last many years—*if* your bite is right and *if* the technician applying them is highly skilled, because the fit is key. If your bite isn't right, your veneers won't last; it's as simple as that. My advice is always to fix your bite first, because I see too many patients who went to other dentists for their veneers, but their bite was not corrected first, and they wound up having to have repairs done.

Recently, I saw a patient who'd had sixteen veneers done but hadn't taken care of them and had not had his bite corrected. They were chipped and cracking, partly because he had bruxism (teeth grinding). I was able to help him out, but the first step was to get that bite corrected, because veneers just aren't engineered to withstand that kind of pressure. Why invest all that money in your appearance just to undermine it with a bad bite? Saving money by not correcting a bad bite may seem to be a reasonable economic decision, but it comes back to bite you.

Crowns

If you've had a root canal done, or you have a genetic dysfunction, or tetracycline staining, a crown may be the only way to repair that tooth. Veneers are thin, and while they can cover some degree of discoloration, the staining can show through if it's extreme.

Invisalign

I love this technology because it treats so many different issues so effectively. Not only can Invisalign aligners straighten your teeth and improve your bite but they also help with clenching and grinding. The fact they're removable means you can still brush and floss without any problems, and of course, since you're solving the problem rather than simply masking it, as you do with veneers, you never have to worry about replacing anything (as long as you wear your retainer).

Receding Gums

Pinhole gum rejuvenation is a great way to add back twenty years to your teeth. With aging, there are receding gums that can be fixed with a "gum lift" —and without sutures and little discomfort. The procedure uses collagen that is added in between teeth with special instruments. Over a six-week period, your body incorporates the collagen and rebuilds gum tissue.

Routine Cleanings

Coming in for a routine cleaning is going to leave your teeth looking and feeling better because we buff the teeth out, polish them with a special paste I have made in my office, and remove all the stains so your smile is improved. Because getting rid of the bacteria is critical, I recommend more frequent cleanings, especially if you are experiencing hormonal disruptions such as the ones that occur with pregnancy, if you smoke or vape, if you're older, or if you have other health challenges that cause bacterial overgrowth.

Whitening

There are three levels of whitening available. The first is the over-the-counter type you can buy at a drug store, such as whitening strips or paint-on whitening kits. The second is the at-home professional kit, which your dentist customizes for you using bleach trays and prescription-strength gel; you do the process yourself over the course of several days.

In-office whitening is the best, in my experience, because of the dramatic effect you can get over a short period of time. When you use the take-home kit your dentist supplies, or an over-the-counter kit, it takes longer to get the same results. If you want your teeth to be one to two shades lighter, you can use the over-the-counter kit. If you're looking to go two or three shades lighter, or to maintain an in-office whitening, the kit your dentist can supply with whitening gel and a mold of your teeth is probably best. But if you want to make a dramatic change and go from four to eight shades lighter, you can get that done quickly in-office. When we whiten, we open up the tubules, so it's like getting a facial. It gets in deep, going into the inner layers of the teeth. That's why it lasts longer. There are different types of in-office treatments: There's Zoom Whitening and EZ White, all peroxide based. I use Zoom Whitening for the most part, but I also do the in-office EZ White if people have gum recession, because the bleach used can cause pain and long-term sensitivity if you have receding gums. I prefer that product in those cases because I can isolate it on the tooth, and I can control the degree of whitening. With Zoom, I can't control the whitening quite as easily.

If you're looking to lighten things up a bit, try an over-the-counter kit a day or two after your professional cleaning. We've got some gel pens at the office that you simply apply to your teeth, and let the gel set for two minutes. They get a good result if you're not after something dramatic.

Whatever whitening process you use, I always recommend using a remineralization toothpaste afterward to minimize sensitivity.

DoTerra is my preferred brand, but any paste with calcium and phosphate or a fluorinated toothpaste will do the same thing.

You can have that beautiful smile you've always wanted—and you can do it by degrees.

Start with the most conservative method, such as a good cleaning, and talk to your dentist about what you want to accomplish and what your options are. Don't go for a quick fix. Instead, start with the fundamentals and look at longevity and functionality. Applying a veneer is easy compared to a bite correction, but an improved bite is better for you in the long term and will help guarantee that your teeth and smile will last for many years to come.

FAQ on Whitening

Q. What can I do to keep my teeth white?

A. Drink your coffee and kombucha through a straw. Come in for your routine cleanings. Avoid drinking lemon water, because it makes your tooth enamel more porous and thus easier to stain. If you do drink it, or apple cider vinegar, for health reasons, drink those through a straw too. And in your hygiene routine, make sure to floss first and brush your teeth for two minutes. An electric toothbrush is much more effective at removing stains. Rubbing your teeth with coconut oil is a good whitener too.

Q. What's the best way to whiten teeth?

A. The safest and best way is at your dentist's office because home whitening is not without risks. If the solution you're using is too weak, it's not going to be effective. If it's too strong and you're not careful about where you put it, you can do serious damage to your gums. While It's not as effective as professional whitening, you can whiten your teeth at home with activated charcoal, which you can get at a health food store in tablet form. Grind it into a paste and *gently* rub in on your teeth with your finger (don't use a brush; it's too abrasive and can cause damage). Rinse and spit two or three times to get it all off before you brush. Another natural solution is to use coconut ghee. You can rub it on your teeth and it will help naturally whiten teeth.

Q. Are over-the-counter home-whitening kits useful?

A. That depends on how much lighter you want your teeth to be. They can certainly take teeth a few shades whiter, but for really significant results, you need to have it done at your dentist's office.

Your Turn:

- If you had a magic wand, what would you change about your smile?
- Do you like the shape of your teeth?
- Do you like their color?
- When you speak or laugh, do you find yourself hiding your mouth or turning away?
- Socially, does your smile hold you back from interacting with others, from starting conversations, or from laughing?
- Professionally, does your smile hold you back from making presentations to colleagues or clients, from

speaking up in meetings, or from interacting with others at networking events?

- Do you get the feeling (or have you been told) that you have bad breath?

If you're curious, keep reading. If you have some questions, give us a call at 415-433-0119.

CHAPTER SIX

Dental Anxiety

*Dental anxiety—the fear of going to the dentist—*is more common than most people think. Those who suffer from it are often ashamed of their feelings and won't admit to feeling fearful about office visits, but from my observations, most people are anxious about visiting the dentist to some degree. Even I sometimes dread going to the dentist—and I practically live in a dental office! An estimated 9 to 15 percent of people suffer anxiety, so the real issue isn't whether or not you have some degree of anxiety, but where you fall on the scale, and whether it's preventing you from getting needed treatment.[16]

---

16 "What Is Dental Anxiety and Phobia," Colgate, September 18, 2013, https://www. colgate.com/en-us/oral-health/basics/dental-visits/what-is-dental-anxiety-and-phobia.

Where Does Dental Anxiety Come From?

For most people, dental anxiety springs from a bad experience in childhood. Maybe they had a lot of cavities when they were young and had to be strapped down to get the needed work done. Sometimes a dentist has been rough, too impatient to wait for the anesthetics to kick in, or just plain abusive. Those kinds of experiences leave a mark and can color all the patient's interactions with dentists going forward.

Dental anxiety can also spring from other kinds of traumatic experience. Some victims of childhood sexual abuse report heightened levels of anxiety when sitting in the dentist's chair. Claustrophobia can be triggered by having to lean back in the chair when people are clustering over you.

It's important to remember that fear isn't really a bad thing. It's a healthy neurological response to a perceived physical threat and helps us keep ourselves safe from harm. When those red flags go up, our adrenal glands go into action, flooding our systems with adrenaline and preparing us to either run or face our attacker in a fight. Our hearts pump more rapidly and our breathing comes faster as this whole panoply of response to the perceived danger takes over our systems. This is all good if you're facing an angry grizzly bear but less useful if it's keeping you from getting the treatment you need to stay healthy.

Some people are afraid of going to the dentist because they have a very active gag reflex, which means that they're apt to start choking as soon as a dentist or hygienist puts a finger in their mouth. They may have had the experience of vomiting at the dentist's office because of this reflex and don't want a repeat of that. Again, this is the body's way of keeping you safe. It doesn't want you stuffing foreign objects into your mouth, but it's gotten a little overzealous in its desire to protect you. When I come across patients with a really potent gag reflex, I help them train themselves to get over it. I give them some tongue depressors to take home, and I instruct them to put a depressor in their mouth every night and hold it for three seconds before removing it. Each night, they must move the depressor back a little bit further than the night before, just to the edge of real discomfort, and hold it there. We find that when patients do this religiously every night over the course of two or three weeks, they can train themselves to control their urge to gag.

I've talked to patients who were made to feel ashamed of their fears by their previous dentist. If that's been your experience, you need to find a more humane and caring practitioner, because you should never be made to feel foolish or crazy for fearing any kind of negative reaction during dental treatment, especially since you've had the courage to admit such a reaction. The fact is some dentists aren't very nice, or gentle, or empathetic. They do themselves and our profession no favors by being that way, but I like to think that a lot of these old-school, my-way-or-the-highway practitioners are now moving toward retirement and will no longer inflict trauma on any more people.

How We Work with Fearful Patients

In my practice, we're very good at helping even the most fearful patients. In fact, a lot of people who start out with us after having bad experiences elsewhere wind up getting over their anxieties altogether. We're able to offer multiple levels of sedation, for instance, which is really useful for gaggers and those who, otherwise, just wouldn't be able to face treatment.

Generally, when patients tell us they're very anxious and ask for drugs to calm them, we start with nitrous oxide, a gas that helps them relax and is delivered via a mask. It's got the added benefit of wearing off very quickly, which means that the patients can drive themselves home after treatment. The next step would be medication, and our first, mildest choice would be Ativan, which lowers anxiety. The second step up in potency is Triazolam, which I'd compare to something like having two glasses of wine. It puts people into a gentle sleep, which allows us to get their dental work done while they snooze.

If the issue is claustrophobia, we accommodate and reassure the patients and work around their limitations of tolerance. It's so much easier for the patients if we're constantly asking, "Is this okay for you?" or letting them sit up and take a break for a minute if they need to, because a lot of this fear is around relinquishing control, and giving control back to the patient is a way to calm their fears.

The best way to soothe dental anxiety is by building a foundational relationship with the patients, talking through the issues and fears. It helps them realize that despite what's occurred in the past, they're in a safe place and nobody is going to do anything they don't want or that will hurt them. We get them to talk through the genesis of their fear, because in order for fear to be overcome, we have to step into that space of fear and experience it to fully let go of it, and then come back to the present reality, realizing that their past negative experience is not the one they're having right now. It's important to get the mind out of the past and into the present so that instead of living in feelings, we're living in facts and in faith.

Everything about our practice is designed to relax patients, starting from their first phone call to booking an appointment. All patients get a welcome letter with some questions that will help us get to know them better and make us aware of what they need, before they get here. It's all about their experience; it's all about them.

We've found that people cope better with anxiety if they've got some food in their stomachs, so we keep snacks on hand if they've forgotten to eat before they come in. We have vegan smoothies in the office with high protein content, which is really helpful. We have relaxing meditation music they can listen to on our noise-cancelling headphones, because many people report being triggered by the noises of a dental office. We even offer aromatherapy. Warm, lavender and chamomile-scented neck wraps are amazingly comforting because we tend to hold a lot of our tension in our neck and at the base of our brain. Many of our patients use them.

I find that deep breathing is a really useful relaxation technique because it helps center us in the *now*. It's very simple: breathe in slowly for a count of five, hold the breath for a count of five, and then slowly exhale for a count of five. As simple as it is, it really works, and it puts the power to soothe themselves into the patients' hands.

Once patients are settled in the chair and comfortable, we talk them through all of the tools and techniques that we're going to use in their treatment and explain the whole process step by step.

If they're even a little bit sensitive, we use a gentle topical anesthetic on their gums before we do any kind of cleaning work, so there's zero discomfort. We also make sure the type of anesthesia we use has a nominal amount of epinephrine in it. Epinephrine is, basically, what keeps the patient numb, but we just use nominal amounts because epinephrine can trigger that fight-or-flight response that your naturally occurring adrenaline creates. Additionally, when anxious patients are being treated or given anesthesia, there's always someone there to hold their hand because we find it helps patients stay "present."

Sometimes people are really good at masking their fears, too good for their own good, in fact. Angela was one of those. A very successful, pulled-together businesswoman, she sat with me as I went over her postexam plan for treatment and nodded as I explained what she needed to have done to fix a cracked tooth. It all seemed to go just fine, but she cancelled her follow-up appointment, and I didn't hear from her again for two years. Honestly, I thought that I had done something wrong or offended her in some way, but it turned out she was just afraid of getting any dental work done. Finally, the tooth in question broke and that got her in at last. Even though there was no longer any avoiding getting that long-delayed crown, and she knew it, it still took us three hours to get her to settle down into the chair because she was so nervous.

So we fed her first, gave her aromatherapy and time for her body to relax, with noise cancellation headphones, and then anesthetized her. We gave it plenty of time to work because fear makes the anesthesia take longer to work. Yes, it took time to make her comfortable, but we got it done, and we did it without traumatizing her further. When she left, she thanked us for being so understanding and told us that she didn't expect to be nearly so nervous the next time she visited our office. Now, she's a model patient and comes in on a regular basis, a win for everyone concerned.

Men suffer the same anxieties and the same kind of shame at admitting them, which they'll sometimes try to cover up by arguing about whether or not they need dental work and by getting angry.

I always try to talk people with this problem through whatever it was that created it in the first place. I've had a couple of patients who told me that their problem stemmed from a near-drowning experience in their childhood. It's good to get them to talk about it. I lead them through an exercise where we go through the sensory experience that created their trauma: what they saw, felt, or tasted and when and how it occurred. Though it may sound counterintuitive, going through the trauma all over again in detail, getting close to the experience actually helps them separate their now-adult self from that frightened child, and let that bad experience go. I have them reassure themselves — "I'm safe. Everything's going to be okay. Everything's going to be okay" —which helps, neurologically, to combat fear. Some patients find they get comfort and control over these feelings by journaling about the experience.

Another good thing for my phobic patients is that I'm a very fast worker and my patients are often astonished that I can get so much done so quickly and easily that they hardly have time to be anxious!

Fear is controllable once you realize that whatever happened in the past isn't happening now. Unfortunately, if those who are fearful don't take the initiative to come to the dentist on a regular basis, they're liable to wind up, like Angela, with a much bigger problem to be dealt with down the road.

The term *fear* can be seen as the acronym for the words "false evidence appearing real." It's something that lives in your mind—and only in your mind, not in your present reality. By the way, it's okay to cry—really, it is—and vent your anxiety that way if you need to. Nobody will judge you, I promise, and at our office, we always have plenty of tissues on hand.

FAQs on Dental Anxiety

Q. Will I be the worst head case you've ever seen?

A. That's a distinction you'll have to work for! Seriously, I deal with these kinds of things all the time, and I get a lot of patient referrals from formerly phobic patients who persuade their fearful friends to visit my office, so it's very unlikely that you'll be the most fearful I've worked with. But even if you are, we'll get through it together, and you'll leave feeling much, much better than you did when you came in.

Q. What happens if I actually throw up while you're working on me?

A. It's happened—more than once—and it's actually not a big deal, believe it or not. We just clean up and move forward. It doesn't happen often, because when I know that's a problem for you, I can work with you to mitigate it.

Your Turn

- Where are you on the fearfulness spectrum?
  - Not fearful: I have no trouble going to the dentist
  - Mildly fearful: I can deal with it.
  - Moderately fearful: It takes some willpower to get me to the office, but I usually make my regular exams.
  - Highly fearful: I only go in emergencies and avoid regular visits.
- If you are fearful, what are your triggers: sounds, smells, the dental chair?
- Try to remember the first time you felt this way. Don't forget that journaling can be very helpful here. You must fully step into your bad experience to let it go.
  - How old are you in this memory?

- Where are you? What does the place look like?
- Who else is there?
- What sounds do you recall?
- What scents do you recall?
- What were you feeling?
- Use every detail to recall it.
- Take ten deep breaths, get "present," look at your surroundings, and realize you are completely safe and comfortable in your home now.

If you're curious, keep reading. If you have some questions, give us a call at 415-433-0119.

CHAPTER SEVEN

Our Teeth as We Age

I've said it before, but it's worth repeating: we're not built to last indefinitely. Our bodies come in for a fair amount of wear and tear over time, and that goes for our teeth too. While we can't stop that aging process, good oral care can buy us time. Let's talk a little in this chapter about what the aging process looks like when we're discussing teeth.

Infancy and Early Childhood

Our teeth begin to emerge when we're about six months old. Typical problems are knocked out teeth or cracked teeth, due to injury. Children in this age group very often develop habits such as thumb sucking, tongue sucking, or pacifier use, which are likely to have an adverse impact on the way in which their jaw or bite develops. It's a good thing to begin caring for baby teeth early on, brushing gently with a finger brush and no paste when they're infants, and then graduating to a child-sized brush and a little dab of paste. When they're old enough to hold the brush, let them imitate your actions, and go over their brushing job with them.

Sugary or starchy snacks are hard on little teeth, and you don't want your child to develop a painful cavity or lose a baby tooth. Raisins, crackers, or teething biscuits create an ideal environment for the growth of bacteria, so limit or eliminate them. The same goes for fruit juice, especially at night, or soft drinks *any time.* Don't put your baby to bed with a bottle, and if you've nursed, wipe your baby's teeth before bedtime.

It's not too soon for that first dentist visit, because you want your child to feel comfortable at the dentist's office and to learn more about hygiene.

Age Seven to Twelve

Seven is a good age to take your child for a first visit to an orthodontist, because some conditions are much more easily addressed at this age than later on. A jaw that is too narrow, for instance, can be corrected without the surgery this problem may incur later on, when the jaw loses its flexibility and the jaw bones are knit.

Keep your children on track nutritionally: no sugary drinks and limited sweets. Let them assume more responsibility for their brushing but still check to make sure they've done it properly, until the age of eight, because their motor skills may not be quite up to the task until then. An electric toothbrush can help them do a better job and is a good investment at this point.

Early to Late Teen Years

Nutrition is a challenge at this busy age, when kids are running from school to sports to other activities. Help them avoid junk food by keeping healthy snacks such as fresh fruit, raw almonds, and veggies on hand and in their backpacks.

The hormonal changes that these years bring mean that keeping up those good hygiene habits is critical. If your children don't have an electric toothbrush, get them one. Get a water flosser, too, and make sure they know how to use it properly. Most teens aren't great at getting up in the morning, so it's up to you parents to be sure they're making time for brushing. Remind them how important their teeth are to their appearance. The desire to look good is probably taking hold about now!

Keep up with regular dental visits and cleanings, and if there are issues with tooth spacing or crowding, ask your dentist about orthodontics. If your child needs braces, get them despite any protests. Your child will thank you later. Braces work faster in a child's developing mouth than they do in a fully adult mouth.

The Twenties

When you're in your twenties, you're probably at the top of your game, physically, and that goes for your teeth too. Everything looks great, but that's a problem because people in their twenties imagine that perfection is going to last forever, so it's hard to get them to take care of their teeth as they should. They skip cleanings and checkups and they skip flossing. Part of this is probably because most of them don't have dental insurance, and young people in their twenties have so many more appealing ways in which to spend their money than in getting their teeth cleaned. A long weekend in Cabo sounds great, but here's the thing: all those missed cleanings and poor hygiene habits are going to be costly down the line, and when the bill comes due in the form of gum disease, these twenty-somethings are going to wish they listened when their dentist sent them those little reminder messages about dental cleanings. All the whitening strips in the world aren't going to help a cavity or periodontitis.

People with bite issues—a crossbite, for instance—are likely to see some accelerated damage to their teeth in the form of potholes. Yep, I said potholes. These little round dents expose the soft dentin within the tooth when the enamel is breached. This can happen when your bad bite puts pressure on your teeth, or when you make your teeth do things they weren't meant to do, such as biting down on rigid stuff never meant to go into the human mouth—that water bottle top, for instance. Acidic and carbonated drinks—lemon water, orange juice, wine, and soft drinks, for instance—help the damage along via demineralization, which is just what it sounds like. Clenching and grinding just kicks the can down the road. There are things a dentist can do to stop those potholes from turning into cavities, but not if you don't see your dentist.

The Thirties

At this stage of your life, a lot of hormonal changes are starting to gear up, and as we learned in the previous chapter, that makes for changes in your mouth too. The chances of getting gum disease accelerate, particularly if you missed all those cleanings back in the day (I'm talking to all you twenty-somethings). Remember that your thirties are the years when stress catches up to with you. That means you'll be experiencing some new and unwelcome symptoms, including the beginning of a decrease in bone density, blood pressure changes, and changes in your thyroid hormones, among other things. Gut issues also start in your thirties.

As far as your teeth are concerned, cavities and gum disease may develop. Your teeth start changing color, too, thanks to all that tea and red wine. And the chewing and pressure you've been putting on your molars is really beginning to wear your teeth down. Molars are the workhorses of your mouth. They're designed to take about 200 pounds of pressure when you bite down, but even they can't withstand the daily grind forever, and evidence of wear is now showing, worse if your bite isn't what it should be or if it has shifted.

Your daily intake of acidic food and drink (that wine, soda, or lemon water) continues to break down and dissolve the enamel, which is becoming thinner over time, with the risk of cavities increasing as it thins out.

Cracks begin to show on those hardworking teeth. If you've really been brutal or your bite is badly off, your dentist may have seen the start of these cracks when you were in your twenties, but they didn't hurt, so you were fine with that. Now that you're in your thirties, they're getting deeper. Why? Your enamel is a brittle structure, kind of like bone. The cracks start in the outer layer, and, over time, go into the pulp and the nerve tissue.

Typically, in twenty-year-old patients, I see the beginning of a small crack in a tooth. At age thirty-something, it's gotten deeper. Sometimes it's painful or cold or heat sensitive; sometimes it isn't, but left untreated, that tooth will continue to crack and, ultimately, break—and that will hurt.

At this point, you and your dentist have got to look at the underlying causes of the cracks and address them. Ninety-nine percent of the time, it's that bad bite. Sometimes it's a side effect of stress: you're grinding or clenching either during the day or, more commonly, in your sleep. We can usually stop that destruction with a customized mouth guard—and you might want to start thinking about how you cope with stress, and what you can do to lessen yours. Often, grinding is a side effect of the medications you're taking. Those for ADD/ADHD, for instance, are a common cause of grinding. Recreational drugs can cause it too. Whatever is making you grind, you need to get help before your teeth wear down to nubs.

The Forties and Fifties

Hey, remember that cracked tooth you had back when you were twenty, the one your dentist probably told you needed fixing, but you didn't have the time to take care of? Now you're forty, and that crack is about to give way—maybe when you're at a holiday meal or a big business dinner—and split in half. This is not a good thing, but at least it will get you into the dental chair, which you may have been avoiding for a while. At this point, you'll need a crown or, if the damage is really bad, a root canal and possibly an extraction and an implant.

You may notice that your gum line is receding, but because it doesn't really hurt, you don't go to see your dentist. The reason it doesn't hurt is that our nerves get increasingly desensitized over time. Your tooth is made up of three layers: the outer layer of enamel, the inner layer of softer dentin, and the nerve in the middle. That inner layer of dentin starts to become harder, thanks to all the stress put on the tops of the teeth over time. As it hardens, you begin to lose sensation at the gum line, where the gums are pulling up and away as the neck of the tooth starts coming down. Why does this happen? Usually the culprit is overbrushing: people want to do a good job so they put too much elbow grease into the effort and wind up doing damage. When you combine overbrushing with bite issues and the inevitable natural wear and tear, you can start getting a lot of problems.

The other thing that begins to happen about this time is that those old fillings you've had for years start showing wear. If you've had a crown for a while, it may be due for a replacement too. Typically, fillings have a life cycle of two to five years, although a crown can sometimes last as long as twenty years. Of course, it matters which tooth we're talking about. Fillings in grinders' mouths tend to wear away every two years, and crowns in grinders' and crunchers' mouths tend to wear away every five. People with a high risk of cavities sometimes get cavities under their crowns or fillings, which is another issue that will need attention because, again, the problems that present themselves are going to get worse if left untreated.

At this age, you're repairing and/or replacing things, trying to forestall the pain of a breakdown or the loss of a salvageable tooth. As it was when you were younger, the mission here is to hang on to the teeth you have, only, at this age, you're finally taking it a little more seriously. Let's hope that you did your due diligence in your twenties in terms of taking care of your teeth and getting those cleanings, because the bill for neglect is about to come due. That said, there's never a better time than *right now* to start taking great care of your teeth. So partner with your dentist to get the help, treatment, and advice you need.

The Sixties and Beyond

By the time you reach your sixties, if you're like most people, you're on multiple medications for issues such as high blood pressure, thyroid and cholesterol problems, and the other age-related conditions we start to see cropping up about now. One of the most common problems people this age report is dry mouth. This can be caused by medications, by hormone imbalances, or by the natural dying-off of salivary glands. Loss of saliva is a problem because it makes your teeth "sticky." Bacteria adhere more readily to your teeth when you've got dry mouth. Typically, dry mouth can cause bad breath, dry lips, and bleeding gums. You're more apt to get candida infections, traumatic ulcers, or traumatic lesions—and cavities.

What medications are you taking? Some of these can also exacerbate issues such as dry mouth, and hormone function (as discussed in a previous chapter) can also present new issues in an aging mouth. Calcium channel blockers are a common cause of dry mouth, and antiseizure medications can cause puffy gums. Anticholinergic medications, tricyclic antidepressants, sedatives, tranquilizers, antihistamines, antihypertensives, cytotoxins, any Parkinson's disease medications, and cancer medication all can cause dry mouth too.

There are mouth rinses to help counteract dry mouth and xylitol-based chewing gum is really helpful too. And stay hydrated! Sipping water all day is good for you, so invest in a toxin-free water bottle and keep it with you.

Another issue that can come with age is loss of sensation in the mouth. That can keep you from feeling a troubled tooth for longer than is good for you. Patients with this problem sometimes wait too long and wind up needing a root canal when a simpler fix would have worked before. Don't skip those exams, folks!

Your bones and joints change, too, as you age. You may already have some issues in your joints. Arthritis can start earlier but is more common from here on, and manual dexterity suffers. Sore hands or wrists can make it tough to brush and floss and some people will slack off on getting those tasks done properly. If you have not already invested in an electric toothbrush and a Waterpik, this is a good time to do so. Both of these work really well and will help you maintain your teeth with minimal effort. Weakening bones, thanks to osteoporosis, are another common challenge in this phase of life. The jaw weakens and shortens, and the bite can change enough over time to create difficulties in chewing. There's a decrease in muscle, too, so that loss of motor function means you can't really chew as quickly. These are all functional challenges that, over time, can undermine good nutrition.

The teeth naturally darken because the inner layer of the teeth changes color. There's increase in oral cancer at this stage of life. Cancers on the lips are common, particularly for those who've used tobacco over a long period of time. Remember your immune system is able to fight things off for a short period of time, but when that same irritant is present over a longer time, it becomes cancerous. Your immune system isn't what it was in your twenties, and if your life is stressful, that's even more likely to be true now. How you handle your stress at this age really matters. As with most things, the stuff you could bounce back from easily in your twenties is going to take a greater toll on you now. Steam rooms and saunas are helpful at this stage because they stimulate the good genes, and intermittent fasting is a healthy way to go, too, giving your body the time it needs to self-regulate.

If you are developing heart issues, as many people in this demographic are, or your doctor has diagnosed you as prediabetic or at risk for diabetes, you really need to be on top of your oral hygiene and get those twice-yearly cleanings, since gingivitis and periodontitis have been shown to be connected to both heart disease and diabetes. More than one in three adults in the USA is prediabetic. Diabetes decreases blood flow to the gums, which means diabetics can't fight off infection, so gum disease gets even worse. That, plus the increased sugar in the blood, creates a big buffet in your mouth for the bacteria, because if it's in the blood, it's in the saliva too.

You'll read more about the genetics of aging in chapter eight, but here are some things to keep in mind as you consider how to maintain your teeth and overall health as you age. To activate those genes that help you stay young, you need to eat lots of green, leafy vegetables, and high quality protein. Exercise is key too. You should get at least thirty minutes a day. Exercising for an hour a day doubles the benefits. Keep your brain active, so never stop learning new things. Research has shown that taking up a musical instrument in later life greatly benefits the preservation of cognitive functions.[17] Additionally, if you're not sleeping eight hours a day, you're undermining your health.

Last, if you're not living an organic lifestyle, now is a great time to start because all that toxicity in your environment is undermining your health.

Every stage of life has its own challenges, strengths, and weaknesses. The good news about getting older? You probably have more money and more time to devote to yourself and your health than you did when you were in your twenties and getting established, or in your forties and raising a family. Use that time to do the things you need to stay well, and your body will thank you for it. Remember, your teeth are so important to your health as you go forward, so make caring for them a priority as you age.

FAQs on Your Teeth

Q. I'm in my twenties, and it's hard to find the money for regular cleanings. Does it really matter?

A. Yes, because you're laying the foundation for the health of your mouth and your body that will either sustain you or let you down as you age. You need to prioritize and make smart choices now because when "later"

---

17   Brenda Hanna-Pladdy and Alicia MacKay, "The Relation Between Instrumental Musical Activity and Cognitive Aging," *Neuropsychology* 25, no. 3 (May 2011): 378–386, https://doi.org/10.1037/a0021895.

gets here, you're going to be stuck with the bill for that neglect. Going to the gym is great. Long weekends away are great. Having teeth that last you a lifetime is also great. Which do you think is the most important?

Q. How long can I expect my teeth to last?

A. Well-cared for teeth should last you a lifetime. Of course, other factors can affect your oral health, but if you are proactive in caring for your teeth and don't put off maintenance, you're going to have functional teeth for much, much longer—and believe me, that's a big deal. If taken care of, your teeth will outlast you!

Q. But isn't new technology going to mean we can all just get a whole new set of teeth implanted in a few years?

A. Right, while we're cruising along with our personal jetpacks. Seriously, don't count on emerging technology to come to market in your time frame or at a price you can afford. Implants are great, but they're not a cure-all—and they're certainly not inexpensive. Wishful thinking isn't a viable alternative to smart choices.

Your Turn

- Are you banking on your future health?

- Life is full of choices, and so many of them will have an impact on us long after we can even recall having made them! Your health today and how you care for yourself is the foundation your future health will rest on. How does your "health account" stack up?

- How many times a year do you go to your dentist for an exam and a cleaning? If it's less than twice a year, you're shortchanging your future health.

- Has your dentist recommended work you're putting off until it's more convenient or affordable?

- How often do you brush? For how long? How often do you floss? Are these activities becoming more difficult for you?

- Does the condition of your teeth or an uncomfortable bite mean that you avoid foods you should be eating such as crunchy, fresh vegetables and leafy greens?

- Do you find yourself salting or sweetening foods more than you used to? This can be a sign of age as our taste buds begin to fail, and neither salt nor sugar is good for our health.

- How are you dealing proactively with stress in your life?

- How much do you exercise every day?

If you're curious, keep reading.
If you have some questions,
give us a call at 415-433-0119.

CHAPTER EIGHT

Staving Off the Aging Process

When it comes to major trends in medicine, genetics are definitely the flavor of the day, and probably will be for some time. The ever-more-accurate ability of science to unravel the information encoded in our DNA is making it possible to do all kinds of things, from uncovering our family origins to tailoring medications to an individual's genetic makeup for the greatest efficacy.

Most of us don't spend a lot of time thinking about our DNA, other than, maybe, getting our genetic genealogy chart done, because there's a pervasive sense that certain immutable facts about our life and health are written in our genes, and we just have to live with them. Whether it's a tendency to develop breast cancer on Mom's side or a susceptibility to Parkinson's disease in Dad's family, the die is cast, and there's not much we can do about it.

It turns out, however, that many conditions and diseases—even how long we live—are influenced by the choices we make, choices that can either trigger or prevent certain genetic traits from being expressed. Once you understand how those triggers work, you can use the information as if you were reading a book in the Choose Your Own Adventure series rather than seeing it as something written in stone. Our genome is the basic language we're given to work with, but our phenotype allows us to be creative with our story's plot; we can choose how our story turns out.

What Is Epigenetics?

Epigenetics is the emerging science of evidence-based medicine (including dentistry) that shows us how to manipulate the expression of the genetic makeup we're born with, mostly by making changes in our lifestyle. Research into epigenetics began in the 1940s. Researcher Conrad H. Waddington, generally considered to be the father of this field of study, coined the term *epigenetics*. Epigenetic changes happen through *methylation*, a process in which methyl groups attach to the outside of a gene and affect the biochemical signals the gene can or can't receive from the body. Picture barnacles clinging to a seashell or mussels growing on a rock, and you'll get a visual of this methylation process.

It's important to understand that these "barnacles" don't change the underlying DNA itself, but rather, how the cells read that DNA and respond to it. Epigenetic changes are happening in our bodies all the time, driven by age, diet, environment, and so on. Those changes can be small and undetectable, or they can cause cancer, for instance. The more we learn about epigenetics, the more we see that so much of our health and longevity is tied up in how the genes we have are triggered by how we live, and while not everything in our genes is subject to our being able to turn it off or on, much is.

Surprisingly, these aren't tough changes to make; they're as simple as eating right, good sleep, lessening tension, exercising, and limiting our exposure to toxins. The question is what all that healthy-sounding stuff looks like in practice.

Eat, Sleep, Move, Relax, Detox

Diet

A high-protein diet, low in carbohydrates and heavy on veggies (especially those rich in antioxidants and lower in starch) is what to shoot for. For gut health, switch to goat's milk; it contains lactobacillus, a bacteria that helps break down food and keeps your gut healthy.

Healthy fat is a contributor to overall health, too, so don't go "fat-free." A pair of studies revealed what researchers say is the best way to limit your risk of most lifestyle-related diseases: one-third protein, one-third fat and one-third carbohydrates, according to the findings of genetic research studies done by the Norwegian University of Science and Technology (NTNU).[18]

Minimize your consumption of meat—no more than 180 ounces a week—especially toxic grain fed red meats. Avoid processed meat such as sausage, hot dogs, deli meats, and bacon. All of these increase the risk for cardiovascular disease and cancer.

Watch what and how much you drink too. Go with organic wine—red is preferred for health since it contains higher amounts

---

18 Norwegian University of Science and Technology (NTNU), "Feed Your Genes: How Our Genes Respond to the Foods We Eat," press release, ScienceDaily, September 20, 2011, https://www.sciencedaily.com/releases/2011/09/110919073845.htm.

of resveratrol, shown to slow down aging—and not too much of it. Best choices in organic wines include pinot noirs, cabernet from California or New York, Italian sauvignon, Australian syrah, and French burgundy. My rule of thumb is always look for biodynamic and sustainable wines such as Dr. Nammy's Nirvana blend. Cut back on your caffeine intake. Coffee is an antioxidant, it's true, but what kind of coffee you drink matters a lot. Organic coffee is a healthier alternative than most store brands, which are usually tainted with mold. So go with brands that don't have mold, such as Purity and Bulletproof coffees. Go easy on sugars, even the healthy kinds.

What you cook *with* is very important too. I'm a big fan of coconut oil because it's good for nearly everything it touches, and it's a great choice for cooking oil. Even better is MCT oil, made from medium-chain triglycerides, a form of saturated fatty acid that has even more concentrated benefits than coconut oil in decreasing inflammation. Avocado and grape seed oil are wonderful for cooking too. Avoid gluten, grains, and dairy, which also trigger inflammation.

Something that is good for you and which you're probably not getting enough of is collagen, which helps promote bone density, increases your antioxidants, and decreases blood pressure. I love a scoop of collagen latte in coffee. In fact, I serve collagen lattes or teas to my patients. Collagen increases antioxidants, decreases blood pressure, and increases bone density.

Intermittent fasting is great at helping regulate sugar cravings and balancing your hormones.

Sleep

Eight hours of high-quality sleep is necessary to almost everyone. In a later chapter, we'll talk a little bit more about what can go wrong when problems such as sleep apnea interfere with your natural rest. Sleep is when your body catches up with needed repairs and repairs cellular damage. Lack of good sleep can trigger genes that cause inflammation and even the genes associated with dementia and Alzheimer's disease. One study[19] discovered changes in 711 different genes after just one week of the mild sleep deprivation of six hours, as opposed to eight. Six hours of sleep is what most of us are used to getting fairly regularly. If you're shaving an hour or two of sleep off your schedule, or you're sleeping badly, you're hurting yourself.

The ideal sleep environment is in a pitch-black room with no Wi-fi devices, and head raised four to six inches on a pillow to improve your lymphatic circulation. So that means no night lights, clocks, cell phones, kindles, iPads, iWatchs, etc.

Exercise

Exercising (or movement) for twenty to thirty minutes a day helps the body to function properly. If you increase it to one to two hours a day, you double the benefits. Good heart health and circulation, and increased oxygen supply to your body cells mean that your whole body is able to function at its optimal capacity. It's been said that "sitting is the new smoking," and that's not an exaggeration. Exercise gives you better health and a better quality of life too. In a 2014 study reported in *Epigenetics*,[20] scientists had a group of healthy young men and women exercise half of their lower bodies—one leg—over a period of three months. As you'd expect, that regular exercise improved the muscle tone in the leg that they exercised, but

19   Carla S. Möller-Levet et al., "Effects of Insufficient Sleep on Circadian Rhythmicity and Expression Amplitude of the Human Blood Transcriptome," *Proceedings of the National Academy of Sciences of the United States* 110, no. 12 (March 19, 2013): E1132–E1141, https://doi.org/10.1073/pnas.1217154110.

20   M. E. Lindholm et al., "An Integrative Analysis Reveals Coordinated Reprogramming of the Epigenome and the Transcriptome in Human Skeletal Muscle after Training," *Epigenetics* 9, no. 12 (December 2014): 1557–1569, https://doi.org/10.4161/15592294.2014.982445.

more interestingly, the scientists discovered significant changes in the DNA of the muscle cells of the worked-out leg, changing their cellular genetic expression. These were genes that control things such as metabolism, insulin response, and inflammation in muscles, but these changes only occurred in the leg that had been exercised. The genes in the muscle cells of the leg that didn't get worked out had no changes.

Yoga and Tai Chi are both forms of low-impact exercise that reduce stress, improve balance, and create calm. The gentle, dance-like movement of tai chi stretches and strengthens muscles and has been aptly described as "meditation in motion." Most exercises will put our bodies into flexion, so all exercise should end with five to ten minutes of back extension, like lying on an exercise ball. Your back will be forever thankful and so will all your internal organs.

Stress

Stress kills, which is why releasing chronic tension and stress are so critical to our well-being. Stress and tension lower our immune defenses. When we're stressed, our fight-or-flight mechanism kicks in, revving our bodies up and draining our resources. A recent study[21] found that this kind of stress affects the sympathetic nervous system and changes the way genes are activated in our immune cells, leading to the increased expression of genes that cause inflammation. We've already talked about the hazards to our health that inflammation creates, and chronic stress is a big contributor that "flips the switch" in the wrong direction on the genes controlling inflammation. But something as simple as regular meditation practice can help, not only reducing stress but actually "counteracting the harmful genomic

---

21   Nicole D. Powell et al., "Social Stress and Myelopoiesis," *Proceedings of the National Academy of Sciences of the United States* 110, no. 41 (October 2013): 16574–16579, https://doi.org/10.1073/pnas.1310655110.

effects of stress," according to the study's senior author, Dr. Herbert Benson.[22]

The reality of life is that it's stressful! We are all here on this planet with a lot to do and little time to do it. So, it's important to have a positive outlook on stress. Our mental state is critical. If someone believes stress is unmanageable, it will be, however, if someone believes stress is going to be there and they can mitigate it, it actually lowers all the negative impacts we associate with stress like heart disease, cancer, insomnia, etc. Personally, I use the mornings to manage my stress. When I wake up, I meditate for twenty minutes, read for twenty minutes and exercise for twenty minutes. This daily routine keeps me fulfilled before I get to the office and give my full attention to my patients and staff.

Check out the technique of Ujjai breathing. I find ten deep breaths can calm me when I'm stressed. Meditation is a tried and true stress buster. Transcendental meditation is my go-to. For those who want to be guided, I recommend *Getting into the Vortex: Guided Meditations CD and User Guide* by Esther and Jerry Hicks. Even ten to fifteen minutes a day make a huge difference.

My go-to for quick relaxation is a nice hot shower with Dr. Nammy's spa mist. Fifteen minutes and I am calm, clean, and happy. The combination of eucalyptus and lemongrass invigorates my mind body and soul.

Detox

Limit your exposure to environmental toxins. Throw away your household chemical cleaners, synthetic beauty products, and unwholesome foods. There's nothing beautiful about beauty products

---

22 Manoj K. Bhasin et al., "Relaxation Response Induces Temporal Transcriptome Changes in Energy Metabolism, Insulin Secretion, and Inflammatory Pathways," *PLOS One* 12, no. 2 (May 1, 2013): https://doi.org/10.1371/journal.pone.0062817.

loaded with phthalates and sulfates that cause increase estrogen. Some of them even contain traces of lead and mercury. Common toxins are skin lighteners, especially from other countries. Read labels and buy only from reputable and responsible manufacturers. Results of a study done at North Carolina State University show that a very common chemical—BPA—has an impact on gene expression related to sexual differentiation and neurodevelopment in a developing rat brain. What is BPA? It's a chemical found in plastic food containers and those water bottles so many of us are addicted to. The researchers Arambula and Patisaul exposed gestating rats to so-called "safe" levels of BPA, and looked at the brains of their newborn pups. According to the study, they found that "prenatal BPA exposure, even at the lowest levels, changed the expression of numerous hormone receptors including those for androgen, estrogen, oxytocin, and vasopressin in the newborns' amygdala, a brain structure involved in a wide range of stress and emotional behaviors. Oxytocin, for example, is important for affiliation and pair bonding, while vasopressin is involved in stress responses. The changes varied depending upon the sex of the newborn and the amount of exposure. Significantly, disruption of genes critical for synaptic transmission and neurodevelopment were also found to be altered, with females appearing to be more sensitive than males.[23]

Think

Lastly, think. "Lifelong learning" isn't a catchphrase, it's a prescription for hanging on to your brain health. Keep your brain active: do puzzles, play word games, or dip into new computer games such as

---

[23] Sheryl Arambula, Dereje Jima, and Heather Patisaul, "Prenatal Bisphenol A (BPA) Exposure Alters the Transcriptome of the Neonate Rat Amygdala in a Sex-Specific Manner: A CLARITY-BPA Consortium Study," *NeuroToxicology* 65 (March 2018): 207–220, https://doi.org/10.1016/j.neuro.2017.10.005.

"Elevate" that stimulate cognitive activity and keep those neurons firing. "Lifetime intellectual enrichment might delay the onset of cognitive impairment and be used as a successful preventative intervention to reduce the impending dementia epidemic," according to a research team led by Mayo Clinic radiologist Prashanthi Vemuri, who researched the effects of continuing study on aging brains and published the results in the journal *JAMA Neurology*.[24]

Pushing Back against Aging

Why do these practices matter so much as we get older? A number of not-so-great physiological shifts take place as we age. Our muscle tone changes because our muscle's natural mitochondria get tired and start to go to fat. Our brains shrink, decreasing in speed and flexibility. It's a lot harder to learn a language, for instance, after the age of eighteen than it is when you're younger than that, and that's all the more reason to keep trying. We lose testosterone, which tends to make us gain fat. We lose estrogen, which weakens our bones and contributes to hair loss. Our thyroids become more sluggish, slowing our metabolism and sapping our energy. Insulin resistance goes up so our blood sugar increases. In our guts, the good and bad bacteria that need to stay in balance can get out of whack, which lowers our immune systems. Food allergies crop up, and bad estrogen—as opposed to the good estrogen   develops, as does the stress hormone *corticotropin*, which effectively pokes holes in the gut. Your vitamin A absorption goes down, along with your vitamin B absorption. DHEA drops are also great after the age of twenty-five. DHEA is

24   Prashanthi Vemuri et al., "Association of Lifetime Intellectual Enrichment with Cognitive Decline in the Older Population," *JAMA Neurology* 71, no. 8 (August 2014): 1017–1024, https://doi.org/10.1001/jamaneurol.2014.963.

the parent horomone precursor and is the building block to help horomone homestasis.

Genes Critical to the Aging Process

A number of genes play important roles in the aging process, and the recommendations above can determine whether they're turned off or on.

The fatso gene (FTO) controls leptin, the hormone that tells you you're hungry. What you eat can turn it on or off. If you decrease the amount of carbs you eat and increase the amount of fiber, you turn it off and that helps with weight control.

The methylation gene, MTHER, directs your body to produce the enzymes needed to process, for instance, vitamin D, creating amino acids, the building blocks of protein. As we age, methylation doesn't work as well as it did when we were younger, which means we're not processing these needed vitamins for cellular health. The Alzheimer's gene is *apolipoprotein* (APoE), of which we have two different types: APoE-e3 and APoE-e4. They cause our bodies to stop recycling cholesterol properly, increasing the risk of cardiovascular disease. You can turn that gene off with proper diet, exercise, and rest, as outlined above.

BRCA is the gene that's associated with a high risk of breast cancer, and it, too, can be mitigated by a diet rich in vegetables to reduce inflammation, and by not drinking alcohol. The VDR gene is what helps regulate vitamin D, which is crucial to bone health as we age and therefore important to keep active.

Telomeres and Aging

At the end of each strand of our DNA are tiny caps called telomeres, which protect our chromosomes. I've seen them compared to the plastic ends on shoelaces in that telomeres basically keep our genes from "unraveling." The length of your telomeres shortens as you age and offers less protection. Interestingly, the length of these telomeres is related more closely to your biological age than your chronological age because how you live affects the health of the telomeres. The shorter they get, the faster your cells age. The strength of your immune system is also tied to the length of your telomeres. Again, diet, exercise, stress reduction, and healthy weight maintenance have all been shown to help preserve telomere health—and help you age more slowly.

Other important genes that affect how we age are the mTOR, the FOXO3, and the SIRT1 genes, known as the longevity genes. They help mitochondria make energy and can be activated by lifestyle. For example, saunas activate the FOXO3 gene and intermittent fasting turns on the SIRT1 gene.

Smarter Supplements

Whole foods are always better than pills because your body has to break down the pill into a bioavailable form to produce energy. However, your body needs supplements to support the health of your bones and teeth, specifically calcium, magnesium, and vitamin D. A basic multivitamin is a good idea and so is the antioxidant resveratrol, that ingredient found in red wine, as I discussed above, and also sold as a supplement. Alpha lipoic acid is another supplement you'll want to include to repair damaged cells. Ubiquinol is great for heart health. I take four different supplements daily: a multivitamin with iron in it, coconut oil with omega-3s, ubiquinol, and a vitamin D complex that includes calcium and magnesium because our bodies can't properly metabolize vitamin D without them. I also like drinking a spoonful of collagen, and my recipe for an immune boost is a mix of turmeric, dried ginger, a little sugar, and coconut ghee. A little of that every day is great for children and adults. Eating raw nuts—five almonds and five walnuts a day—is also a great health practice.

Healthy Ages and Stages

Children who are a few months old up to eight have an immune system that is a work in progress, so if they're in day care or school, they're going to be exposed to various viruses and bacteria and will bring them home. Boost their immunity with fresh citrus, a multivitamin, and frequent hand washing. Kids are really moldable at this age, so start setting the stage. Start training your kids to have healthy habits, including drinking green juices, and boost their immunity with turmeric and ginger drinks.

Tweens and Teens need lots of positive reinforcement because self-esteem is an issue at this stage. Hormones present physical and emotional challenges, so be aware of your children's changing body and talk to them about it. Make sure they have healthy foods available, and that they're not living on ramen and pizza because "that's all there was." Many girls start on birth control pills, which can cause moodiness and other issues. Hydration and sleep is key. At this stage, teens are very susceptible to self-doubt. So, remember to encourage your children and boost their self-esteem. Help decrease their cortisol levels.

This is a great time to add mindfulness to eating as well as meditation.

Older teens and college-aged kids have more challenges coming at them including drugs and alcohol. Keep the dialogue going and don't judge. They want your input even if they don't ask for it. Bulimia is a problem for many at this age. Your dentist can see the telltale signs in acid damage to their teeth. The good news is that their concern about their appearance can be a reason to eat well and take care of themselves too. This is also a great time to get genetic health testing with 23andMe to get an idea of what optimum health will require.

In our twenties, we're still coasting on the energy of youth, and too often, we're writing checks on our health by not getting the regular health care we need. Many who developed suboptimal eating habits in college or high school continue to take poor care of themselves. Most important at this stage is to eat vegetables and exercise thirty minutes a day!

The thirties, forties and fifties see perimenopause. For women it begins around the age of thirty-five. For men, it begins at about the age of fifty. Many systemic conditions start manifesting at around the age of forty, such as high blood pressure, diabetes, and COPD. If your work is sedentary, make time for exercise and de-stressing. Its time to start intermittent fasting and using a sauna twice a week. Hydration, and balanced sleep and exercise are crucial at this time. Add in calcium, magnesium, and a vitamin supplement to help manage stress. Start tai chi to increase bone density.

In the sixties and seventies, dry mouth becomes a problem. We don't have the energy we had even in our forties, and one problem—such as high blood pressure—leads to another, such as diabetes. Alzheimer's and dementia begin to show up. Tooth loss becomes a problem too. Start using substitute saliva. Eat lots of veggies.

FAQs on the Aging Process

Q. If I eat a healthy diet, do I really need supplements?

A. In an ideal world, we'd eat a perfectly balanced diet every day and our systems wouldn't be under attack by environmental toxins. We'd get adequate sunshine, and we'd never overdo it on coffee or wine. But most of us live in a world where meals are too often grab and go or left out altogether. There's no good reason to skip supplements; they exist to help us fill in those nutritional gaps and support cellular health.

Q. If my family tends to be long-lived, doesn't that mean that I'm more likely to be?

A. Generally speaking, yes, but the choices you make in terms of diet, exercise, and so on are going to have a big impact on not only the length of your life but also the quality of your health during your life. That's why it's important to be aware of how your own practices affect your genetic makeup; you want to celebrate your one hundredth birthday feeling great.

Q. I've read that some people can sleep as few as four hours and still be healthy.

A. It's possible for a very few, thanks to a genetic anomaly uncovered in a 2009 study[25] led by Dr. Ying-Hui Fu, a neurology professor at the University of California, San Francisco. She mapped the genomes of a patient who, as did the rest of her family, reported feeling well rested after just four hours of sleep, and found that they all shared a mutation of the gene DEC2. This gene mutation was not present in the family members who slept longer. Dr. Fu reports that she's subsequently encountered only a few hundred people with this mutation that allows them to sleep so little, yet remain healthy and energetic. Some people, she says, train themselves to become short sleepers, but it's not natural or healthy for them, even if it becomes habitual, and they're more likely to experience adverse health effects.

Your Turn

Rate your health habits: grade yourself 1 for "Yes", 2 for "Most of the time," and 3 for "Almost never."

1. I am careful about the quality and quantity of what I eat. My diet is rich in organic leafy greens and antioxidant vegetables and fruits, and light on red meat and grain.

2. I usually get seven to eight hours of sleep a night.

3. I exercise a minimum of thirty minutes a day.

---

25 Ying He et al., "The Transcriptional Repressor DEC2 Regulates Sleep Length in Mammals," *Science* 325, no. 5942 (August 14, 2009): 866–870, https://doi.org/10.1126/science.1174443.

4.   I make time to de-stress: to meditate, take a long hot bath or sauna, walk in the woods, do yoga—whatever calming activity works for me—daily.

5.   I'm careful about how much alcohol and coffee I drink and limit myself to one glass/one cup a day.

6.   Supplements are a part of my daily routine.

Score:

6–10: You're doing very well.

11–15: Good work! Now move toward improving those areas for which you scored less than 1.

16–21: You are putting your health at risk. Make the changes now that can help you roll back the damage and enjoy a long and vigorous life.

If you're curious, keep reading.
If you have some questions,
give us a call at 415-433-0119.

CHAPTER NINE

The Importance of a Healthy Bite

Let me tell you about Julie. She was twenty-six when I met her. She had a wonderful smile, thanks to orthodontics, and a fast-paced career in tech, with all the attendant stress. But her smile wasn't much in evidence when she told me about her problems with jaw pain and headaches. An exam uncovered the symptoms of clenching and grinding, and also of the probable underlying cause: a malocclusion (better known as a bad bite).

Shown the evidence, she was astonished; she'd just had her teeth straightened a couple of years previously, so how could her bite be bad? I had to explain that there was more to healthy tooth placement than appearance. I designed a set of aligners to deal with this underlying problem, and three months later, her jaw pain was gone, and her clenching and grinding had decreased significantly.

Elsewhere in this book, I've talked about the evidence supporting the many advantages enjoyed by people with beautiful smiles, from overall happiness throughout life to self-confidence, career advancement, and social interactions. But there's another aspect to the placement of your teeth that's not nearly as obvious, yet arguably even more important to your oral and overall health. That's your bite, and even a pretty smile doesn't guarantee that your bite is as healthy as it needs to be. The worst of it is that you may not even be aware of the problems your unhealthy bite is causing you.

Orthodontics and periodontics together are the cornerstones of good dental health, and they have been mostly ignored for too long. If your gums aren't healthy or your teeth properly aligned, your oral health will suffer even if you look good. The bottom line is that when your bite is out of alignment, it's got to be fixed through orthodontics because no matter how great your teeth look, function is more important than cosmetics, and it will come back to bite you if you let it go.

Let's start with *headaches.* Did you know that over 80 percent of headaches come from issues with the jaw and the bite?[26] It's strange but true that a misaligned bite stresses the muscles of the jaw and causes spasms that create headaches. When teeth don't mesh properly, they strike each other with more force than they should, and that repeated impact can also create a tension headache.

TMJ and Head/Jaw Pain

The *temporomandibular joint* (TMJ) of your jaw can also cause pain that can radiate through your head. This joint works like a

---

26   "Study Suggests Tension Headache May Actually Be TMJD," University of Buffalo, Science Daily, May 14, 2006, www.sciencedaily.com/releases/2006/05/060514082537. htm.

hinge connecting your jaw to your skull. Many things can cause TMJ problems to develop at different points in life. The joint can be knocked out of whack by an injury, or stiffen up because of arthritis. Very often, habitual grinding or clenching causes these TMJ problems. When you grind your teeth, you do so with extraordinary force. Ordinary pressure for a bite is about 175 PSIs, but the pressure from grinding can get up to 500 PSIs. This is likely to do damage over time, but it's exacerbated when your bite is out of alignment and can cause TMJ pain.

Signs of a TMJ problem include:

- a clicking or grating noise when you open or close your mouth,

- pain in the joint, especially when you chew,

- radiating facial or head pain,

- frequent headaches, and/or

- pain or difficulty in opening or closing your mouth.

None of the fixes you do for your teeth—not veneers, not the work accomplished by braces or aligners, not even your fillings or crowns—will last if the bite's not right. The bite is not just about the teeth. It's about the way that the jaws fit together. It's about the muscles. It's all about form and function.

A Surprising Major Cause of Bad Bites

Among people who've had braces, one of the biggest causes of bad bites is that orthodontists in the past simply moved teeth too fast. This ended up creating a lot of TMJ damage. Now we do functional orthodontics in that we strive to align the bite, the jaw joints, and the muscle so there's no extreme stress on the bite.

In correcting these issues, my preferred system is Invisalign, clear aligners that move the teeth. I go with a specific protocol in my practice that's a little different from that of some other practitioners because we've found it decreases allergic reaction. Our aligners are cleaned with distilled water, and are hand cut versus laser cut. I also move the teeth really slowly to minimize resorption (which is when the tooth starts dying on its own), and to avoid TMJ damage. I don't recommend any other brands because they contain bisphenol A (BPA), a cancer-causing agent.

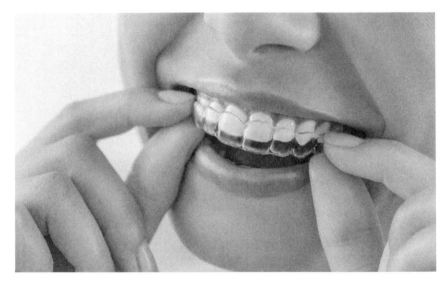

Aligners have the additional benefit of helping with clenching and grinding because they're like a pillow between the teeth and will make clenching and grinding painful, especially during waking hours. The pain creates a negative feedback loop, making patients aware of their habit and thus helping to break it. I see about an 80 percent reduction in clenching and grinding among my patients using aligners.

How Do I Know If My Bite's Off?

Even if you started life with a healthy bite, our teeth shift as we age, so spacing changes. Braces also change things, and not always for the better. Alternatively, you may have had your teeth moved to a good bite position but then neglected to wear your retainers.

Think of the tires on your car. They've got to be replaced regularly because friction wears them down and reduces the tread. The same kind of wear happens to your teeth. Your mouth gets used a lot! You use it to chew all the time, and when you're clenching/grinding, you're using it on overdrive. Some of us drive our cars more than others do. I've only got thirty thousand miles on my car, but I have friends who drive 150 miles a day, so their tires get replaced pretty often because there's more wear and tear. Your teeth wear faster if you clench and grind.

One warning sign that usually develops over about ten years of stress on your teeth are cracks. All that pressure put on them is more than they're built to endure. You might also notice that the metal in your fillings is brighter where it's being worn down, or that you can see metal showing through your crowns.

You may spot little potholes in your teeth, where the outer layer of enamel has been worn down and the inner layer of the tooth is exposed. These are a real concern and need to be attended to.

A bad bite causes abfraction lesions (bruises at the root surfaces). These form because of the great pressure from the top of the teeth, and they create a sort of growing "notch" that cuts into the tooth structure just at or below the gum line. The neck of the tooth eventually becomes so narrow that it fractures off. These abfractions are also caused by stress, in the sense of high pressure on the tooth. If you're seeing these notches at the gum line and are noticing that your teeth are getting more sensitive, you need to see your dentist.

But My Orthodontist Told Me My Bite Was Fine …

Like what happened to the patient I talked about earlier in this chapter, teeth do relapse—and the relapse starts immediately. If you had orthodontia as a kid, it doesn't mean your mouth—and consequently your bite—stopped changing and growing. Your muscles and skeleton continue to develop and mature after your braces come off.

Did you hang on to your retainer, or lose it and neglect to get another one? That's the most common reason teeth slide out of alignment. There's no "safe" period in which you can stop using your retainer, though people often make that mistake. Your teeth will move if you don't use it.

If you've been told you have a bad bite, or if you suspect that you do, please don't put off seeing someone who can assess that for you. While it's not necessarily even visible to the untrained eye, I promise you that the problems it will cause you down the line will be only too easy to spot—and to feel!

FAQs on Bites

Q. Why are my lower front teeth showing signs of wear?

A. That can be symptomatic of a bad bite because they're rubbing against your upper front teeth in a way they're not supposed to. You're probably seeing the dentin, the layer that's under the enamel, and that dentin isn't nearly as hard as the enamel that's supposed to be there to protect it, so the damage is going to get worse, faster.

Q. When I clench my teeth, some of them hurt. Why is that?

A. A bad bite, typically, puts extra pressure, and a lot of it, on a few teeth, which causes both pain and damage. These teeth may, eventually, crack under the strain. If they're crowns, they'll have to be replaced because they'll be damaged. If you're a nighttime grinder or clencher—a lot of people are but don't know it—it will happen faster. Get it checked.

Q. I suddenly have a sharp pain just in front of the hinge of my jaw when I eat. How could I have TMJ problems develop so fast?

A. It may seem sudden, but in fact is more likely to be a problem that's developed over time without your being aware of it. That said, jaw problems can be caused by even a minor injury to the face, something you might have brushed off at the time because nothing seemed hurt. In any case, please get it assessed because TMJ can create so many problems.

Your Turn
How's Your Bite?

- Is eating causing you any discomfort? Do you find it difficult to bite into food or to chew it without pain?

- Do you hear a clicking sound when you open or close your mouth?

- Does opening your mouth wide cause pain in your jaw hinge?

- Do your jaws and/or teeth ache when you wake up in the morning?

- Do the clench test: clamp your teeth together with nothing in your mouth. Do you feel any pain in any of your teeth? Is there no contact between some of your teeth, or extra pressure on some others?
- Do you see cracks forming in any of your teeth?
- Are there rough spots on your teeth, or on your fillings?

If the answer to any of these questions is yes, please see your dentist and have your bite assessed or give us a call at 415-433-0119

CHAPTER TEN

"But Why Does Treatment Have to Cost so Much?"

Recently, a new patient told me he'd been to another dentist three months previously but was concerned about his long-term oral health since he didn't think that previous cleaning had gone deep enough. I agreed to take a look. The x-rays revealed that he had significant deposits of calculus. I took gum measurements and found five- to six-millimeter pockets, which were bleeding. In addition to all of this, his bite was off. I told him he needed a deep cleaning.

I pointed out several problems that his previous dentist hadn't mentioned to him: cracked teeth, a worn-out crown, old amalgam fillings that had been in his mouth for years and that were starting to crack. He had a cross-bite, too, and those potholes I've mentioned. All of these problems needed to be addressed. Worst of all, his previous dentist had done a deep cleaning and left radiographic calculus behind. Yikes!

He agreed to the treatment. He signed the consent form that outlined all his costs. Then he sat in the chair and numbed up. The cleaning took over two hours, using the laser tool to disinfect his gums. Subsequently, we repeated the x-rays to make sure that we'd located and removed all that calculus and tartar that his previous dentist had left to harden. It was a thorough job and he left in much better shape than when he had arrived.

When he got home, he called us to argue about the bill. He'd signed a consent form, which clearly stated the costs. He said he didn't remember, so I sent him a copy, along with a detailed description of all the work we'd done in that hour and a half he'd been in the chair. Clearly, this man had a problem with money or trust. I am interested in working with people who want to take care of their teeth, so they can chew properly, be comfortable, and look good. Our values did not align. So, I wrote off his account and said goodbye. The fact is I do what I do because I love it. We did great work and he just didn't appreciate it. It was clear this man was looking for free services and he was distrustful.

It's important to look at the facts concerning your gums and your teeth. Yes, there are always more appealing places to put your money: a vacation, or a car, or a designer bag. When you're talking about your health, however, price should be the last thing on your mind because the only person who is accountable here is you. I'm always proactive in recommending fixing the bite and healing ailing gums first, but as the saying goes, you can lead a horse to water (and even show him the x-rays), but you can't make him drink. So sometimes, even long-term patients decide against getting their bite corrected, and wind up with so many more problems, and so much more expenses.

So many people simply put off needed work on their teeth, most often because of the expense involved, but that falls into the category of a false economy because, as is true in almost every other area, just ignoring a thing doesn't make it go away. Would you ignore a "check engine" light on your car's dashboard or a lump on your body? Of course not. You'd call the mechanic or be in the doctor's office the next day. And though you might not relish the expense, you'd figure out a way to pay and be grateful to have it taken care of.

Dentistry is no different; and although it may seem costly, it costs money for me to house, to staff, and to supply my practice. The materials we use are very expensive, as are the tools. A single laser wire is $800. My license has to be renewed annually for $800. My insurance is over $2,400. We pay hefty city taxes and all the other expenses associated with renting. The continued training I take is expensive too. I'm all about doing the best possible job for my patients and getting them from wherever their neglect of their health has left them to the best, most hygienic and functional place possible.

While I can do a lot to improve my patients' conditions, the fact is, they have to be accountable for their share of minding their health. They have to eat right, exercise, stick to their daily oral hygiene routines—all the topics I discuss in this book. Patients with periodontal disease have to face that fact and deal with the consequences caused by neglect. I'll do my part, but I can't be responsible for what a patient does or does not do outside my office. Yet I'm sometimes challenged by patients to justify the expense of treatment they didn't even know they needed until they came to me for problems far more extensive than they imagined they had.

We Make It Easier to Handle Costs

We get it: People don't usually have piles of money sitting in their back accounts that they're able to drop on dentistry. Emergencies come up, dental and otherwise, and many of us have so many competing claims on those same dollars that it's tough to know where to put them. But I believe very strongly that my patients deserve the very best care, and we've come up with solutions to make that possible, even for those whose budgets are stretched.

For instance, we offer interest-free financing for twenty-four months; we pick up the interest charges and the patient gets the services. We do that as a courtesy for our patients because we're sincere in our desire to get them well and keep them that way. That said, it's still frustrating to me when a patient whom I've been telling for years to take care of an issue while it's still minor puts off treatment until the issue becomes major and then blames me for the cost of repairs. If I tell a patient, "Your tooth has a crack in it, and your bite is to blame," I make it clear that within three or five years, it's going to break. If I tell patients they've got serious periodontal issues that are undermining their teeth and that, in time, they're going to lose their teeth because of the periodontitis, and they shrug it off, they pay the price in the years to come.

Their attitude reminds me of the way in which so many people view their eventual retirement. We all know that, inevitably, there will be a day when we'll have to depend on our savings and whatever other provisions we've made for income, in lieu of what we made while working. It's common sense, and as predictable as the sunset, but how many of us take it seriously enough to plan for it? The figures are daunting when you look at how few people have made or are making the proper financial preparations. It's like a time bomb, ticking away in our economy—and all because of a lack of personal accountability and the magical thinking that if they just put it off, somehow it'll take care of itself. That doesn't happen with your teeth any more than it does with retirement planning.

We give our patients a comprehensive treatment plan because that's what practitioners with integrity do. We let patients know from the get-go what the work they want will cost. Some of my patients, who have access to that kind of cash or are ready to talk about financing, say, "Go ahead," while others choose to proceed a tooth or two at a time.

Another new patient, a young woman with a mouth full of old amalgam fillings, asked me to remove all the mercury from her mouth. I examined her, and told her it would cost $20,000 to remove all the mercury fillings, but we didn't have to do them all at once. Her response was outrage. She couldn't see past the quoted price to what I was trying to do, which was to fully inform her and present her with options to get her where she wanted to go.

People aren't always ready to go ahead, and that's okay. We simply do the work they're comfortable with, at the pace they want; it's really about serving my patients and helping them in the best way I know how. My feeling is always that if we can get started with work at that initial visit, it's going to save those patients the bother of an extra trip to the office, but if they're not ready to proceed, for whatever reason, all they need to do is to voice that concern. It's all about being transparent. At my practice, if finances are a problem for patients, they should tell me so that we can come up with a solution that will get them where they want to go at a price they can afford.

Be accountable about your needs because, as in any relationship, you need to make sure you're communicating.

The patient I mentioned above will probably go to another dentist and say, "Hey, my last dentist told me I needed twenty grand's worth of work done, and I don't want to do that." Do you think the other dentist is going to say that she needs twenty grand's worth of work? No, he's going to tell her she's just fine, and "Let's just get this cleaning done, and then phase your work in a little at a time." It's like dating. If, on that first date, you tell your date, "I want children," how likely is it that person will be honest with you about having children? What you will hear is: "I am open to having children with the right person."

Trust between Doctor and Patient

Therese is a long-term patient of mine, and a great example. When she came to me several years ago, her teeth were in awful shape. Much of it was genetic; some of it was bad oral care. In her forties she had already lost teeth, and she was ready to take comprehensive steps to fix what was wrong. After her initial exam, we had a long talk about what I saw as a treatment plan. She needed six front crowns, and a couple of implants. Her bite was off too. I told her straight that it was going to cost $50,000 to get all of that fixed, but we didn't need to tackle it all at once. Based on that conversation and her own instincts, she decided to trust me. I told her, "Okay, let's do step one, which is the crowns on your front teeth. Once that's done we can go to step number two, which is the implants. Once that's done we can go to step number three to make sure that you're comfortable and your bite is functional."

It took time, but we got through it, and she's a loyal and grateful patient who comes in every three months for cleanings—and yes, it was expensive, but losing teeth is worse.

And the news isn't always bad! Some people, particularly those who feel guilty about having gone too long without seeing a dentist, come in expecting to have to pay much more than they actually do. It's a pleasure to be able to tell them that the cost to fix what's gone wrong is going to be much less than they had anticipated. And sometimes genetics are on your side! Amazingly, some of these folks don't need more than a cleaning to get back on track.

FAQs on Dental Treatment

Q. I'm getting different messages from different dentists about what I need. Who can I believe?

A. Trust is difficult, but be sure not to confuse trust with fear of cost. It can be confusing and overwhelming, especially if we're asked to choose between courses of treatment when, as consumers, we're not really well informed. Do your due diligence and ask questions. If a dentist makes a recommendation, ask to see the evidence that supports that recommendation, including x-rays, research articles, scans. The dentist should answer all your questions patiently, fully, and without hesitation. If you suspect that he or she is telling you what you want to hear to spare you sticker shock, ask about that too!

Q. My course of treatment is really expensive, and I'm worried about how to pay for it.

A. Your dentist should offer you some options. Maybe, all of that work doesn't need to be done all at once. Sometimes we have to "triage" our patients, and help them see what is really pressing versus what can wait. Ask about that: what must be done now versus what could be put off? Ask, too, about financing. If your dentist doesn't offer what we offer, find out how he or she *can* help. Some dentists will give you a break if you pay cash, for instance. In some cases, health savings accounts can also be utilized.

Your Turn

- What are your personal priorities? We "feed" what matters to us: with money, with time, with attention. Take a few moments and consider where your spending habits suggest your priorities are, and consider, too, if they're where they should be.

- Are any of the following statements true or false for you?

    □ I live within my means, and don't struggle with debt. If I can't afford it, I don't buy it.

    □ I would rather have a vacation than healthy teeth.

    □ My car says more about me than my smile.

    □ I regularly put money away for retirement, even though it sometimes means I have to miss out on things I want, because the future matters to me.

    □ My retirement plan is, basically, suicide.

    □ I love buying designer shoes because I know that people seeing them will "get" that I'm successful. They won't judge me because of my health, but by my appearance, so Jimmy Choos are a better investment for me and give me more pleasure.

- I look good right now, and that's good enough for me. Why spend money on something I might not really need when there are things I want?

- Dentists are mostly shysters, anyhow. They just want to upsell you on stuff you don't really need.

Now think about your responses. What do they say about your ability to plan thoughtfully for the future? What kind of steward of your health are you?

If you're curious, keep reading. If you have some questions, give us a call at 415-433-0119.

CHAPTER ELEVEN

Dental Materials and Technology

In other sections of this book, I've touched on some of the materials commonly used in dentistry today. I think the topic bears a lengthier examination, especially for those of my readers who are concerned about what is put into their mouths and what the long-term effects of those materials can be on their health. If you're not, maybe you should be!

I think everyone who gets dental care needs to be aware of the choices that are out there, and why some are demonstrably better than others. After all, it's your body, and you're paying for this work, so why not be a better-informed consumer? Not all dentists will be this forthcoming about materials, and those who aren't holistic in their clinical orientation may not be as knowledgeable on the topic, so this chapter is here to help you understand what kinds of questions to ask about treatment options.

We'll start with the *metal materials* because these are the ones I'm most often asked about in my practice.

Generally, I'm not a fan of metals. I don't use amalgam fillings at all in my practice (see chapter three) and I prefer to minimize the use of metals in general. Some people have sensitivities to metals, and if you suspect you're one of them, you should have compatibility testing before you have them put into your mouth. Typical allergies we find are to nickel, beryllium, cadmium, and mercury. It's also best to avoid palladium and silver because they have been found to cause sensitivity in eczema patients.[27] Corrosion is another concern. Pure gold is great, but who can afford it? Mixed metals, on the other hand, harbor bacteria. If you have a crown built on a metal base, the metal and those bacteria can contribute to inflammation.

Porcelain is what we typically use, and my favorite is E-MAX, which is manufactured from *lithium desilicated ceramic*. It's durable, translucent, and can be made to fit better than metal-based crowns, plus you run nearly no risk of allergic reaction because it's 99 percent compatible. It's great for back teeth because it's as durable as a natural tooth structure and looks natural in place. Its durability is a big strong point over previous generations of porcelain crowns, which generally wear down faster than the neighboring natural teeth. If the crown is too strong, on the other hand, it will cause your natural, opposing tooth to wear down faster, so a match in durability is the ideal.

Composite Fillings

The replacement for amalgam fillings is made of composite, which is composed of rocky silica particles held together by a batter that

---

27   Werner Aberer et al., "Palladium in Dental Alloys: The Dermatologists' Responsibility to Warn?" *Contact Dermatitis* 28, no. 3 (March 1993): 163–165, https://doi.org/10.1111/j.1600-0536.1993.tb03379.x.

hardens when it's "cured." The cure is done via exposure to UV light. It has three components: a filler, a monomer, and an initiator. The filler is porous and can be lithium, aluminum, silicate, barium, or strontium. It's held together by this soupy mix called BIS-GMA, which is made with BPA. We talked about the dangers of BPA in a previous chapter, but just to refresh your memory, these are plastics used in food containers and water bottles and they can leach into the water or food. BPA mimics estrogen in the body, and because certain estrogens can cause cancer, BPA adds to that risk. Composites, however, are made not to leech, by adding a *glycidyl methacrylate* that stops that from happening.

Composites are a terrific alternative to amalgam. Their application is technique-sensitive, but if they're done right, they're both durable and attractive.

Indirect Restoration: Onlays and Crowns

An *onlay* is made from either porcelain or gold and is cemented on a tooth that requires partial replacement. You can think of it as a halfway solution that falls between a filling and a crown.

A *crown* covers the whole tooth, not just a section of it. When decay or damage has taken away more than two thirds of a tooth's structure, the remedy is a crown.

In my practice, we make crowns for back teeth right here in the office, using a specialized 3D printer. This has a lot of advantages for the patient, including not having to go home with a temporary crown, and not having to come back for a second appointment (or get a second shot, for that matter). Another upside is that it's the best process for your mouth in that it doesn't create as much inflammation, because the tooth and the nerve are healed in a single process. Every time we work on a tooth, it's going to get irritated and inflamed, so less contact is better when you're talking about the healing process. Think of having a scab, and how much longer it takes for the wound under it to heal if that scab gets knocked off. It's like the process has to start all over again.

We can do a great job of color matching, too, and people are delighted with the results. When it comes to front teeth, though, I send that work out to a lab because the more translucent material they use to make them is prettier.

Our goal is always to conserve the tooth structures. I don't take the margins (the bottom) of the crown underneath the gum tissue, as many dentists do, because we're able to color match so nicely. I leave it on top of the gum because it's easier to clean, which means less bacteria, and the material lasts longer.

Implants

Implants are far from a new idea. In fact, the first implants we know of were bits of shell, implanted in the mouth of a Mayan woman in AD 600, and the ancient Egyptians also used shell and pieces of polished bone to replace teeth.[28]

The science behind modern implants is based on a discovery of a Swedish researcher in orthopedic surgery, Dr. Per-Ingvar Brånemark, who was studying how blood flow affects bone healing. He implanted tiny cameras encased in titanium into the leg bones of rabbits to observe the healing process, but when his research team tried to remove those devices, they discovered that the titanium casings had fused to the bone. Brånemark immediately saw the potential for

---

28   Celeste M. Abraham, "A Brief Historical Perspective on Dental Implants, Their Surface Coatings and Treatments," *The Open Dentistry Journal* 12, no. 8 (May 2014): 50–55, https://doi.org/10.2174/1874210601408010050.

dental implants that would fuse with the jawbone, and called that process "osseointegration."

That process is why my preference is always for implants over less permanent solutions such as bridges. Implants actually help the jaw regenerate bone, which is especially valuable as we age and our bones start dying. Missing teeth in the jaw make the bone even more vulnerable and weak, and an implant can turn that process around.

Between porcelain implants, zirconium and titanium implants, my preference is for the latter because porcelain fails faster and tends to fracture. My favorite product in this category is Nobel Biocare Active, a titanium implant. It's inert, which means that it has no chemical reaction with the body. The bone grows around it perfectly and it lasts the longest that I've seen in the industry. A titanium implant creates a stable and lasting tooth, and is a better investment over the long term than a bridge, which is guaranteed to fail. There are a few ceramic options that I use. So far, I have done about 7,500 titanium implants, and they're doing great.

When we're planning an implant, the first step is to get a CT scan, and figure out the density of the bone. We try to minimize the number of implants that we have to place. Once they are placed, we have to wait three months before the procedure is finalized. You still have a tooth during that process.

Sometimes a bone graft is needed if a tooth has been missing for a long time, because the body has been eating away at the bone in that area. Usually, a bit of cadaver bone is packed into the area, and it actually beefs up the strength of the bone in that area. We're very scrupulous about cleaning the implants with ozone or oxygen before we place them, to kill bad bacteria.

There's so much about bridges to dislike. First, you can't clean properly between the teeth, so you're much more likely to get gum disease and a cavity underneath the tooth, which will most likely lead to tooth loss, and a root canal if you haven't already had one. Removable partial dentures have their own limitations. Among other things, they're not stable, and interfere with speech and (often) eating. To me, the whole idea of bridges and dentures feels pretty last century. When science has evolved so much, why are we still doing things the same old, nonoptimal way? The cost of implants has come down substantively in recent years, and they're also far more comfortable and easier for the dentist to do well.

Lasers

The first laser was built in 1960 by Theodore H. Maiman at Hughes Research Laboratories. It was based on earlier work by Charles Hard Townes and Arthur Leonard Schawlow and their device, which was dubbed the maser. That name itself is an acronym for light amplification by the stimulated emission of radiation. What seemed like science fiction when it was introduced is everywhere now, from supermarket scanners to cat toys—and your dentist's office.

Basically, two types of lasers are used in dentistry: cold and hot. Cold lasers are set at a wavelength of about 650 to 800 and are what we typically use on the gums to photostimulate them. The photon emits packets of energy and light which are absorbed by the gums' cells, so they're energized to heal. They make energy called ATP (*adenosine triphosphate*), which feeds the cellular function, decreasing pain and inflammation and promoting healing. These kinds of lasers have many applications. They can be used to speed healing on cold sores, to decrease gum sensitivity or postsurgical pain, and to kill bacteria lurking in the gums next to the bone. To some degree, they also stimulate bone growth in halting the inflammatory process and promoting healing.

Especially for people who tend to get a lot of tartar and plaque, including diabetics, hypertension patients, or patients going through hormone therapy, decreasing the bacteria in their mouths is very helpful. When patients have a higher degree of gum disease, we use laser therapy to disinfect the pocket and promote healing. Laser therapy requires the practitioner to make a sizeable investment. The laser itself costs from $10,000 to $50,000, the training to use it runs about $3,000, and the fibers it requires are about $800 apiece. You can see why dentistry costs what it does. No thoughtful practitioner wants to be without up-to-date tools and technology, and while that doesn't mean chasing every shiny object that comes along, it does require significant and ongoing financial investment to make sure patients get what they expect: the most advanced and most effective level of care.

What's the Story with Fluoride?

The use of fluoride is controversial because fluoride displaces the iodine that is needed for proper thyroid function. I do use fluoride in my practice. I don't recommend it for everyone, but if I had to choose between having a cavity or using fluoride, my choice would be fluoride because cavities are worse for us than fluoride is. In my practice we're careful to control where the fluoride goes when it's administered so that it's absorbed only in a localized area rather than through the whole body. The problems you hear about are related to systemic fluoride.

FAQs on Dental Technology

Q. Can anyone get dental implants?

A. As long as you've got healthy gums and the underlying bone isn't beyond repair, you should be a good candidate for implants.

Q. Does having an implant mean I don't have to brush that tooth?

A. No. Keeping the implant and the area around it clean are absolutely required for the health of your mouth.

Q. I wanted implants a few years ago, but they were pretty expensive, and my insurance wouldn't cover them. Is that still the case?

A. Prices have gone down a lot in the last few years, and many insurers are now covering at least part of the cost, so it might be time to revisit that option. The other thing to remember when you're weighing the cost of an implant is that a titanium implant done right will outlast anything else you can put in your mouth, and that means no retreatment or replacement costs down the line. Plus, it looks and feels like a natural tooth, and no bridge will ever feel as comfortable or be as easy to clean.

Your Turn

If you're in the process of choosing a dentist, here are some questions you ought to ask your prospective practitioner:

1. **Do you use dental lasers for cleaning?** While the standard cleaning procedure a hygienist performs is

still part of a good cleaning, a dental laser accomplishes so much more beyond simply removing plaque and tartar, and it's really the standard of care you should demand because the bacteria it destroys are the greatest danger to your oral health.

2. **Do you use amalgam fillings?** Believe it or not, there are still dentists out there who do—lots of them. If you're going to a dentist who uses amalgam fillings, that's an indicator that he or she is behind the times and not taking a holistic view of health.

3. **Do you do biocompatibility tests for materials?** Before placing metals in a patient's mouth, your dentist should offer to test for allergies.

4. **Do you use digital x-rays?** They are far more accurate, faster, and lower in radiation than the old-style x-rays.

5. **Do you make crowns in your office, or send them out to a lab?** If your dentist can't create a crown for you in her or his office, that means an extra visit—maybe even a third if your temporary crown falls out—more time in the chair, more anesthetic, and so on. More of everything except convenience!

If you're curious, keep reading. If you have some questions, give us a call at 415-433-0119.

CHAPTER TWELVE

Creating a Healthy Oral Environment

I've talked in earlier chapters about nutrition and how it contributes to (or diminishes) both your overall health and oral health. In this chapter, I'll focus a little more narrowly on the oral environment itself and how what you put into your body affects it.

The pH of the Mouth

A major piece of creating a healthy oral ecosystem is maintaining the proper pH of the mouth. Just to be clear, pH is the scale on which we categorize the relative acidity versus alkalinity of a substance. Pure water has a pH of 7; anything that falls below that is higher in acid, and anything above 7 is more alkaline. Battery acid (sulfuric acid) has a pH of zero; antacids have a pH of 11.

The ideal pH level in the mouth is about 7, like blood, which registers at 7.5. Anything much lower than 6.5 and that acid environment is going to begin to eat away at your teeth. *Acidemia* is the proper name for a high-acid oral environment, and that can happen to your mouth in a number of ways. First, it can come from what you eat and drink: soda, lemon water, apple cider vinegar, or any citrus, even wine. Just make sure you rinse thoroughly after consuming anything high in acid.

Chronic inflammation causes an increase in *monocalcium*, which leaches calcium out of the teeth and the bone. The peptide hormone *angiotensin*, created and released by the liver as the protein *angiotensinogen*, is broken up by enzymes in the kidney to form angiotensin, which causes an increase in calcium in the blood. That calcium is pulled out of bone and teeth, weakening them.

Oxidative stress, which has been linked to multiple serious health issues, happens when there are too many *free radicals* floating around.[29] Free radicals are molecules released in chemical reactions. The antioxidants we consume grab those free radicals, deactivate them, and get them out of our systems, usually. But when that free radical is hyperactive, oxidative stress can occur. Mercury in your system increases oxidative stress. Any heavy metals will do that, which is another reason not to put them in your mouth.

Acid in the mouth increases the amount of tartar. It will cause cavities and gum disease because those bacteria grow best in acidic environments. Acid in the mouth also comes from stomach problems or inflamed intestines, celiac disease, and from leaky gut.

---

29   Bayani Uttara et al., "Oxidative Stress and Neurodegenerative Diseases: A Review of Upstream and Downstream Antioxidant Therapeutic Options," *Current Neuropharmacology* 7, no. 1 (March 2009): 65–74, https://doi.org/10.2174/157015909787602823.

What Is Leaky Gut?

Intestines are normally semipermeable in that certain materials such as nutrients can pass through a healthy gut and into your body, but a healthy gut also maintains a barrier to keep potentially dangerous things from migrating out into the body. Our bodies have many barriers, starting with our skin, that are there to protect us from harmful substances. Leaky gut, though, means that damage to the lining of the small intestine allows various toxic waste products, food particles, and bacteria to leak into the body, causing all kinds of problems, among which are food allergies and yeast infections. When other kinds of imbalances are added to the mix—such as mercury or hormone issues—they increase the problems with food allergies and the candida fungus.

So how do we get that desirable pH balance in our mouth? Start with getting rid of, or at least radically decreasing, your intake of refined sugars. Real fruit is a great source of healthy sugar. Fructose and corn syrup, on the other hand, are awful. Xylitol is one that I would recommend as well; agave and honey are also healthy, though agave is processed. I recommend coconut or brown sugar to my patients over white processed sugar, but even these should be used in moderation.

Avoid toothpastes that contain sodium lauryl sulfate (SLS). This causes the oral mucin layer, the membrane lining the inside your mouth, to slough off, which can cause *aphthous ulcers,* those nasty little spots better known as canker sores. Tricolsan should also be avoided as well as artificial color and sweeteners. I would definitely avoid fluoridated toothpastes for kids and women with thyroid issues.

Another great way to help the pH balance in your body is to drink warm water with a few drops of lemon juice in it. Drink it through a straw, though! Even though the lemon is acidic, once in your body, it helps to normalize your acid balance. Another helpful thing is chlorophyll water, which is made with a few drops of concentrated chlorophyll added to water. Leafy greens help balance your body. Apple cider vinegar is great for digestion too. I would make sure you drink it through a straw!

A healthy alkaline diet calls for us to increase our intake of lean protein, decrease our intake of carbs, and eat more good fat. Keeping a healthy balance of cholesterol is important, because it supports healthy hormone production, which in turn protects your body from certain cancers. Cholesterol-lowering drugs can create an imbalance that actually raises your cancer risk, which is another reason I advocate using a healthy diet and lifestyle to regulate those numbers. Natural is best: healthy diet, rest, exercise—all of these things will help to regulate your body. That goes for supplements too; you're better off eating an orange than taking a vitamin C pill.

Dos and Don'ts for a Healthy Oral pH Balance:

- Do sip sodas and acidic drinks through a straw to minimize their contact with the teeth and tissues of the mouth

- Don't brush your teeth right after drinking acidic drinks (including wine), or fruit juice, because the acid has softened the enamel and brushing while it's still soft will do damage. Instead, chew some sugarless gum containing Xylitol to encourage salivation, which will help to remove the acid and rebalance the pH of your mouth.

- Do drink plenty of fresh, clean water during and between meals. It helps your whole body and also aids in keeping your teeth clean and your mouth hydrated.

Testing and Analysis

One way to find out whether or not you're in balance is to do analyses or tests of various kinds. I don't do many of these tests. I send my patients who wish to have them to naturopaths to administer them. They can include

- Tests on hair

- Blood tests

- Urine and/or fecal analyses

When we do a hair analysis, we're looking at thyroid function by checking the calcium levels we find in the hair. A higher-than-normal level of calcium present in the hair could indicate a sluggish thyroid. A decrease in potassium means that the thyroxine cells are not responding. Typically, we want a four to one ratio, with four parts calcium to one part potassium. Again, a higher calcium ratio than that is potentially a sign of hypothyroidism.

We're also checking for zinc and copper. Too much copper can cause alopecia and hair loss, as well as arthritis, mood swings, and acne, as the immune system is weakened. Too much zinc in your system means your collagen functions are going to be impaired and can lead to anemia and osteoporosis. A higher-than-normal potassium count points to issues with the adrenal glands; if you have low potassium, you won't be able to produce cortisol, which is critical to health because it takes glycogen and turns it into glucose, which is a stored form of sugar. If you're short on cortisol, your body won't be able to turn its stored fat into energy when it needs to. If you don't have that energy function, your immune system suffers, and you're more likely to suffer from allergies and from adrenal exhaustion because your body is on overdrive.

Aldosterone is a *mineralocorticoid* found in hair. A high level of aldosterone increases the sodium levels in your hair, which points to acute stress and potential adrenal burnout. An increase in sodium levels and in the sodium to potassium ratio tells you that the thyroid gland is not working and there's acute stress. An increase in potassium means chronic inflammation. Your hair can also be tested for heavy metals, especially for mercury toxicity.

I've talked a lot about the kinds of bacteria that can cause gum disease, and we test for those right here. We do the BANA test, which checks your tongue coatings (*subgingival plaque*), for a trio of bacteria associated with gum disease and bad breath: *Porphyromonas gingivalis, Treponema denticola*, and *Bacteroides forsythus*.

FAQs on Healthy Oral Environments

Q. What's the best kind of dental floss?

A. I always recommend coco floss because it has coconut in it; coconut happens to be a natural astringent. I prefer waxed floss for comfort and ease of use.

Q. Does it matter what kind of toothbrush I use?

A. I recommend an electric toothbrush because it's going to do a better job than hand brushing. The brand I like is Oral B; it's actually got an app that lets you share your brushing history with your dentist. If there's some gum recession going on, I recommend something called the Rotodent. Its bristles are really soft and it helps keep the gums comfortable and not over-brushed. It's a gentler kind of toothbrush.

Q. What kind of mouthwash should I use for my breath?

A. Generally, I don't like mouthwashes because they contain alcohol, and really, the only thing they accomplish is to make you feel fresh. If you're concerned about your breath, your best bet is to get in the habit of scraping and brushing your tongue as part of your regular oral hygiene practice. That will certainly do more for your breath than any rinse.

Q. I've still got my wisdom teeth. I've been told I should get them taken out, but they don't bother me, so why should I?

A. Dentists generally promote the removal of wisdom teeth because they are a potential source of infection. If a tooth is half exposed, food gets stuck in there, creating a perfect environment for gum disease and inflammation to take hold because the chances are good you're not really brushing it well since it's so far back in the mouth. You're making your body work harder than it should to keep that inflammation under control and maintain your health. So why keep the tooth that's really no use to you?

Your Turn

How's Your Oral pH?

I drink water ...

1. When I think of it

2. When I'm thirsty

3. All day, every day

I eat sugars ...

1. Of all kinds; sugar is sugar

2. On a limited basis, and am careful about what kinds of sugar I consume

3. Primarily in the form of fresh fruit

My food intake is mostly ...

1. Whatever I can grab

2. I watch what I eat, but it's not always optimal.

3. Lean protein, limited carbs, plenty of lower-starch vegetables, and healthy fats

Reader, if your answers aren't all 3s, you haven't been paying attention. Being mindful about what goes into your body is part of being a good steward of your health.

**If you're curious, keep reading.
If you have some questions,
give us a call at 415-433-0119.**

CHAPTER THIRTEEN

Sleep Apnea in Adults and Children

Snoring, long the subject of jokes, complaints, and—mostly ineffective—over-the-counter remedies, may seem like an odd topic for a book on dentistry, but thanks to modern technology and a new understanding of what makes us snore, and its effect on our overall health, snoring is getting more serious attention. Not everyone who snores has sleep apnea. Snoring can be symptomatic of allergies, for instance, or temporary and caused by a cold or other upper respiratory viruses. But chronic snoring is one of the signs of apnea, and apnea is no joking matter.

There are three types of apnea:

- **Obstructive sleep apnea**, caused by the relaxation of the muscles in the throat and tongue or by the presence of enlarged tonsils or adenoids

- **Central sleep apnea**, a disorder caused by your nervous system, when the brain fails to send the proper signals during sleep to the muscles that control breathing

- **Complex sleep apnea syndrome**, which is a combination of both obstructive and central sleep apnea

Why is sleep apnea a big deal? Because we're seeing that apnea is related to a whole range of long-term health problems that go far beyond its most obvious symptom, which is daytime sleepiness. The problems include heart disease, diabetes, and stroke, among others.[30] One in five adults suffers from sleep apnea.

What Are the Most Common Symptoms of Apnea?

- The above-mentioned daytime sleepiness is one. Do you usually get up feeling less than rested, even if you've had what should have been a full night's sleep?

- Does your partner tell you that you snore?

- Do you wake yourself up with your snoring?

- Does your partner report that you occasionally stop breathing and gasp for breath before settling back into sleep?

- Do you have difficulty concentrating?

- Are you irritable?

---

30   Jean-Louis Girardin et al., "Obstructive Sleep Apnea and Cardiovascular Disease: Role of the Metabolic Syndrome and Its Components," *Journal of Clinical Sleep Medicine* 4, no. 3 (June 15, 2008): 261–272, https://www.ncbi.nlm.nih.gov/pmc/articles/PMC2546461/.

- Have you gained weight or do you find it difficult to lose weight?

- Is your blood sugar level rising?

- Do you find yourself getting tired or even nodding off during the day, especially while driving?

- Do you often wake up with a headache?

- Do your jaws and teeth ache in the mornings? This can be caused by a number of things, including clenching and grinding, but it can also be symptomatic of apnea, since the body is straining to try to correct the improper breathing.

- Do you have GERD or acid reflux?

- Do you depend on stimulants such as coffee and energy drinks to stay awake?

- Is your tongue "scalloped" around the edges? This is a sign we look for when apnea is suspected.

- Do you have a thick neck? A large neck circumference— more than forty-two centimeters, for instance—is an indicator.

Obesity is often the cause of apnea, but you don't have to be obese to suffer from apnea, and apnea itself can contribute to obesity. It can also be caused by drinking alcohol, but not always.

Our bodies need oxygen to function, and apnea cuts it off. Problems such as heart disease, obesity, and cognitive impairment occur because we need oxygen and we're not getting it.

How Can Your Dentist Help?

If you suspect you have apnea, your first visit should be to your doctor, and your second to your dentist. While removal of tonsils and adenoids can often cure apnea, other issues can also create apnea such as a too-small jaw. Your dentist may be able to recommend ways to treat it nonsurgically—for instance, with an oral appliance that effectively pulls the tongue forward. There's also a newer therapy called Inspire that uses an app to turn on a small remote control device that activates the sleeper's hypoglossal nerves to tell the tongue to keep its tone, so it doesn't fall back into the throat.

If you suspect you may snore, there's also an app that helps you check your snore cycle. It's called SnoreLab and it's a good way to find out how much you're snoring and how often. If you do snore, the next step is that doctor visit and exam, and potentially, some sleep testing in a lab.

Apnea in Children

Believe it or not, children get apnea too, and because their bodies and brains are developing and growing, the physical toll on them can be even more devastating. Yet their symptoms and signs don't necessarily present themselves in the same way as those of adults, and that can keep them from getting properly diagnosed and treated.

In fact, researchers are finding that many children who have been diagnosed with ADD/ADHD are actually undiagnosed apnea sufferers.[31] As it turns out, what causes sleepiness and low energy in adults can have the opposite effect on children, who will present what

---

31   Louise M. O'Brien et al., "Sleep and Neurobehavioral Characteristics of 5- to 7-Year-Old Children with Parentally Reported Symptoms of Attention-Deficit/Hyperactivity Disorder," *Pediatrics* 111, no. 3 (March 2003): 554–563, https://doi.org/10.1542/peds.111.3.554.

looks like hyperactivity and overstimulation as a result of chronically broken sleep.

If you suspect your child has apnea, or if your child has been diagnosed with ADD/ADHD, you need to be aware of the signs of apnea in children:

Does your child ...

- Snore loudly?

- Toss and turn during sleep, or sleep in odd positions?

- Wet the bed after having previously been dry at night?

- Snort or gasp during sleep?

- Get teased at slumber parties for snoring?

- Show increased irritability, moodiness, or daytime sleepiness?

- Have trouble concentrating in class?

- Have behavioral problems at home or at school?

- Have difficulty catching his/her breath when participating in sports?

If any of these symptoms are present, your child may have apnea and should be tested. A too-narrow jaw can be the problem, and if it's caught early enough, expanders can be used to treat it while the jaw itself is still flexible and growing. If the problem is tonsils and adenoids, or allergies, these are easily treated, too, and can make all the difference in your growing child's health now and in the future.

FAQs on Sleep Apnea

Q. I snore when I've got a cold. Is that apnea?

A. More than likely, if you only snore occasionally, it's not. But if you suspect—or your partner suspects—you snore when you're not congested, talk to your doctor and your dentist about it. Better safe than sorry.

Q. If I'm overweight, will losing the weight stop the snoring?

A. If excess weight is the underlying cause of your apnea, then most likely, losing weight will solve your problem, and in any case, you'll be healthier than you are now! But if the snoring persists, please get checked for other issues, because apnea does contribute to continued obesity and the inability to keep weight off, along with all its other harmful effects.

Q. What about sewing a tennis ball into the back of a sleep shirt to keep me from sleeping on my back as a remedy for snoring?

A. You're right in thinking back sleeping is a contributor. People who sleep on their backs are twice as likely to snore and have apnea. Sleeping on your left side is, generally, the best position from the point of view of health. But if there's an underlying problem causing the apnea, your sleeping position isn't much of a solution, so you should still bring it up with your doctor and dentist.

Your Turn

Apnea can be a killer, literally, yet many people don't realize they've got it.

1. Do you wake yourself up snoring, or does your partner tell you that you snore?

2. Are you overweight?

3. Are you a restless sleeper?

4. Are you groggy during the day?

5. Are you forgetful?

6. Do you have difficulty concentrating, or a sense of mental dullness?

7. Do you need a lot of coffee or other stimulants during the day to keep yourself going?

8. Have you ever either fallen asleep at the wheel or "zoned out" while driving?

9. Is your tongue scalloped around the edges?

If you answer yes to one or more of these questions, you may be at risk for sleep apnea. Please see your doctor and your dentist for help and proper diagnosis.

If you have some questions, give us a call at 415-433-0119.

CLOSING THOUGHTS

Does your dentist have a mission? That may sound like an odd question to ask, but consider this; how we see ourselves in life, particularly as health care practitioners, has a huge impact on how you, as a patient, are seen and treated, whether that's as a name in an appointment slot, or as an individual worthy of care and respect.

I have a mission, and a vision. Simply stated, the vision of my practice is to create an open and inviting atmosphere where we grow lifelong relationships with both our patients and team. We are a community of environmentally conscious professionals and leaders; we offer our patients the best resources, technology, and services to provide dental health with the highest standards. *We are caring people caring for people.*

Most of all, we educate and empower our clients to bring the best of systemic health to their lives, and that is the purpose of this book: to help people live longer, healthier, and more joyful lives. That's why this book is about so much more than "drill and fill." Everything you do, everything you eat, all the choices you make are tied together and affect your health—and why wouldn't you want to enjoy the best possible health for the longest time?

As far as we know, we just get this one life. I believe that each of us should do our best to live that life to the fullest, but what I see so often is otherwise intelligent people who think short-term—this week, this month, this year—and that's just not good enough. We really need to start looking at ten years, fifteen years, twenty years or fifty years out and investing our intelligence into researching what it takes to live not just longer but better.

Did you know that between the ages of twenty and fifty, people lose seven to ten permanent teeth, on average? About 10 percent of Americans between the ages of fifty and sixty-four have no teeth left.[32] Those teeth didn't just all fall out one morning. A lifetime of neglect went into their loss. It's like having a little leak in your roof: do you stick a bucket under it, or do you get it repaired properly? You know what happens if you choose the bucket route. Sooner or later, your roof is going to fall in.

I've said it a few times in this book but it bears repeating: life is brief and we're not built to last indefinitely. That said, we *can* enjoy the process of maturation if we're prepared for it. A lot of the assumptions we make about aging are based on how we saw our parents or our grandparents live. Those things aren't necessarily true for us. We know now that our genes aren't our destiny; advances in epigenetics are letting us take our futures into our hands and change it, not just play the cards we're dealt. Surviving is good, but surviving and thriving is better.

My practice is a welcoming practice. From the moment you call us, you can expect the best possible service and care from everyone

---

32   "Tooth Loss in Adults (Age 20 to 64)," National Institute of Dental and Craniofacial Research, last modified July 2018, https://www.nidcr.nih.gov/research/data-statistics/tooth-loss/adults.

you come in contact with. We care about you and your values and we care about your health and your comfort. We know that having you as a patient is both an honor and a sacred trust, and we strive in every way to serve you as you wish to be served. You can also expect to leave knowing more than you did when you came in; not just about your specific needs but also about health and wellness in general. I see our relationship as a partnership. I welcome your questions, your concerns, and encourage you to learn more and be a better advocate for your own health.

Beyond the walls of my office, my advocacy and support for health extends globally. At this writing, I am creating a nonprofit dental clinic in the Indian village my family came from so that children and adults there will have access to the care they need. I've named it in honor of my late brother, and it's a heart-centered mission for me. Why? It's not that I needed one more thing to do, I promise you, but I want to leave a lasting and meaningful legacy. I want the world to be a better place because I have lived in it. I want to share the good fortune I've had, and the knowledge I've accumulated with those who are less lucky than I've been.

Being a caring person who cares for people is at the heart of my mission, and I hope that if you're within reach of our practice, you'll give me the opportunity to share that caring with you.

At Green Dentistry, we're invested in the latest advancements in high-tech dentistry and promise to enhance your visit with relaxing, luxurious spa-like amenities. We specialize in holistic, functional dentistry and offer many general, cosmetic, and restorative services, including:

- gum disease treatment
- root canals
- sedation dentistry
- dental implants
- crowns
- veneers
- pinhole gum rejuvenation
- and much more!

To schedule your appointment,
visit www.sfgreendentist.com,
or call us at 415-433-0119.

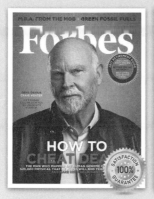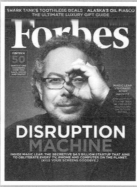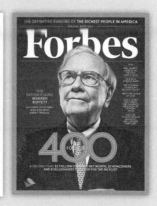